VITAMIN O

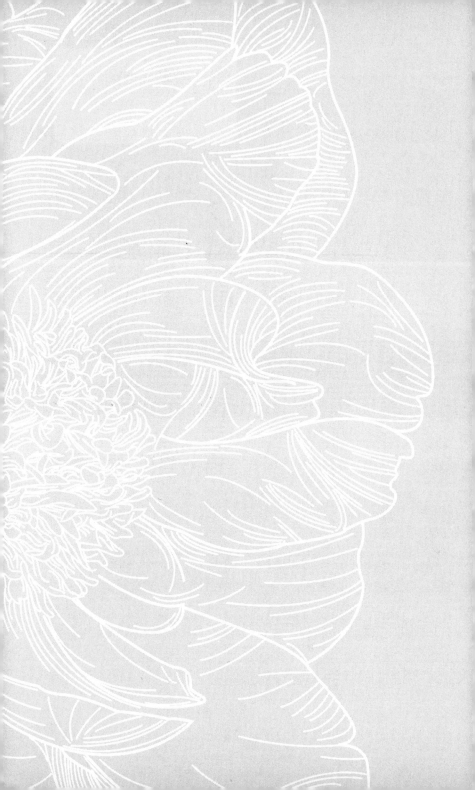

VITAMIN O

WHY *orgasms* ARE VITAL TO A
WOMAN'S *health* AND *happiness*—AND
how TO HAVE THEM *every* TIME!

DR. NATASHA JANINA VALDEZ

CLINICAL SEXOLOGIST AND AUTHOR OF *A LITTLE BIT KINKY*

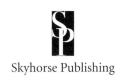

Skyhorse Publishing

Skyhorse Publishing books may be purchased in bulk at special discounts for sales promotion, corporate gifts, fund-raising, or educational purposes. Special editions can also be created to specifications. For details, contact the Special Sales Department, Skyhorse Publishing, 307 West 36th Street, 11th Floor, New York, NY 10018 or info@skyhorsepublishing.com.

Skyhorse® and Skyhorse Publishing® are registered trademarks of Skyhorse Publishing, Inc.®, a Delaware corporation.

www.skyhorsepublishing.com

10 9 8 7 6 5 4 3 2 1

Library of Congress Cataloging-in-Publication Data is available on file.
ISBN: 978-1-61608-311-3

Printed in the United States of America

To every woman on the planet but especially
my girlfriends Mariska and Blaire. You were the
inspiration for this book.

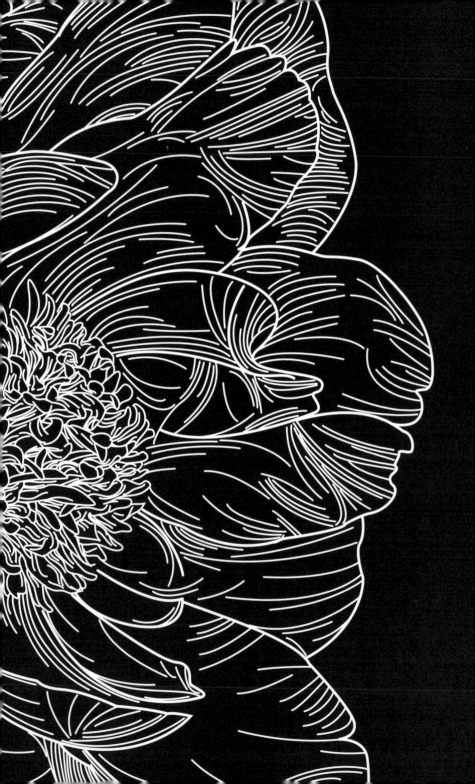

CONTENTS

HELLO, MAGIC *O*!

"An orgasm a day keeps the doctor away."
—MAE WEST

What if I told you there was a vitamin you could take that would enhance your mood and your lifestyle? That would curb your appetite and lower your cholesterol? That could drastically diminish your risk of heart disease and stroke and boost your immunity? That could recharge your relationship? And then, on top of all this, it had no adverse side effects, was absolutely free, fun, and even kind of yummy—and you didn't have to swallow it? Well guess what?

There is, it will, it can, it doesn't, and it is. And you can get it in my most favorite way.

Introducing VITAMIN O, a revolutionary, yet not-so-new, life-enhancing "supplement" that nourishes body, mind, and soul—and it's created right in your own body! The O stands for Orgasm. The Vitamin, for all the benefits this "magic tingle" provides. When you incorporate regular doses of Vitamin O into your life, you'll be amazed how everything improves, from your performance at work to the way you cope with stress to your very outlook on life.

In my experience as a clinical sexologist, I have discovered that one of the most common sex issues women face is not being able to have orgasms—or have ones that really satisfy them (No, there is no such thing as a "bad" orgasm, but there surely are degrees of good!). Through the years, both in my private one-on-one sessions and with listeners of my former radio show and viewers of my TV appearances, I've helped thousands of women have better orgasms than they ever dreamed possible with more frequency than they ever imagined. Now, with Vitamin O, I'm going to share my secrets with you.

This book is a book about orgasms—and orgasms for women. (Sorry, men, but this is not something you guys typically struggle with.) In order to have better orgasms and more of them, we're going to get to know them inside and out. We're going to discover the potency, and then we're going to show you (and your partner) how to unleash their power for yourself.

We'll begin discussing Vitamin O by delving into the science behind the orgasm: what an orgasm is and what it does to your *whole* body. Don't skip over it—it's short, I promise! You're going to get a lesson about orgasms you'll never forget. After that, we'll get into all the great benefits this amazing Vitamin provides. And then after we talk about all the wonderful "ayes," we'll quickly get into the "nays"—namely, what are some of the reasons you're not having the orgasms you should be having, and start finding ways back to getting them. I'll even introduce you to some of my clients who have worked through many of these common issues.

After class comes the fun part: the action! In *A Little Bit Kinky*, I showed you tons of fun and playful ways to reconnect with your partner. When it comes to orgasm, connection is key for women, I'll give you plenty more of these suggestions and activities here. We'll get acquainted with our own bodies, and we'll learn how to express with our partners what makes us feel good. Then we'll explore all the manual techniques, oral methods, and crazy-fun sex positions that maximize your pleasure. I'll show you how to have a variety of orgasms (it's not just about the clitoris, ladies), and because there are so many types of releases, it increases the likelihood you'll have orgasms, by yourself or with a partner. Health-boosting, life-affirming orgasms—and in ways you've never considered.

We'll cover the basics in orgasmic foreplay, orgasmic positions, exercises to improve orgasms, orgasm-enhancing yoga, breathing techniques, and more. We'll even get into more advanced climaxing—multiples and simultaneous orgasms. Look for my "quick fixes" throughout the book to help you get your daily dosage of Vitamin O without any fuss.

By the time I'm through with you, having orgasms will become as natural and pleasantly habitual for you as drinking your morning coffee (which, because you'll be sleeping better and have more energy, you'll be drinking less and less of). You'll be healthier, you'll be heartier—and you'll be a heck of a lot happier. And there isn't a single vitamin on the shelf that can guarantee all of that!

—Dr. Natasha

VITAMIN O

disc*O*

pOi

r the

ency

Not every pleasant indulgence in life is bad for you. Not everything that makes you feel like you've gotten away with something good is wrong or dangerous. Sometimes a "guilty pleasure" is just what you need to be enjoying—and without the guilt, ladies! Of course, everyone knows that orgasms feel good, but let's find out what they're all about and why having them is so healthy for you.

CHAPTER 1

THE
SCIENCE
OF BLISS

"Electric flesh-arrows . . . traversing the body. A rainbow of color strikes the eyelids. A foam of music falls over the ears. It is the gong of the orgasm."
—ANAIS NIN

A h, the orgasm. That electrifying tingle that awakens our senses, pumps us up with all kinds of good feelings, and makes us feel truly alive like nothing else. Anais Nin, a famous erotic writer, explains it pretty well, I think. But there is so much more going on in an orgasm than just plain "magic." Because yes, it is a magical thing, but there's real science behind all those "arrows" and "rainbows" and the "foam of music" Anais describes.

In this brief chapter, we'll walk through just what is an orgasm, what happens to your body when you have an orgasm, what does an orgasm feel like, and how does it make you feel. The last part of this is no mystery for those of us who have experienced orgasms—and good ones. But if you belong to the group of women who feel like they've never had an orgasm before, or if you're not really sure if you ever have, this chapter will take away any doubt. And for those who determine they've never had an orgasm, it will leave them with a sense of delicious anticipation.

ONE EQUATION, *many* PARTS

So what exactly is an orgasm? In the most basic terms, it's a release of sexual tension. Orgasm in men is marked by the release of semen—not exactly something easy to fake. For women, orgasm is a mostly internal process of pleasant muscle contractions that take place in rapid succession, some less than a second apart, in the pelvic region. (By the way, ladies: The female orgasm is also not exactly something that's as easy to fake as you think it might be—but we'll get into why people do fake orgasms, why you really actually can't, and in fact never should a bit later.)

Now there's been some debate on whether or not orgasms are felt the same way in both women and men, and the short answer is that they are indeed similar—though not the same. In each, an orgasm is a quick series of pelvic contractions, in the genital and anal regions, about an eighth of a second apart. The good news for women is that ours can be much more intense as our uteruses may also contract (and in a pleasant way), which means more areas affected and deeper within us. Of course, for both sexes, orgasms are pretty much triggered the same way: through stimulation, sometimes physical, sometimes not.

> In her book, *The Case of the Female Orgasm*, Dr. Elizabeth Lloyd says women are less likely than men to be tired after orgasm. Which explains why your partner pretty much passes out afterward, and you feel ready to pop out of bed and paint the bedroom!

So orgasms are never exactly the same. They can be felt differently, by both women and men, in terms of how powerful they are, how long they last, and how intense they are. This all has to do with a number of factors, including excitement level, how much time has passed between orgasms, how much energy the one being pleasured has at the time of stimulation—and how little energy. So there's a lot past "the mood" that goes into having orgasms—and having good orgasms.

Of course, the orgasm is just the grand finale. To take full advantage of Vitamin O, we also have to look at how to get to that final destination. The parts of the equation are as important as the sum because if the parts don't add up correctly, the equation just won't work.

Okay, so what are the "parts?" For the purposes of this chapter, we're just going to talk about parts of your body that are important to orgasm and how it all comes together—in other words, the physiology of the orgasm. We'll get into the emotional component—and the actual "doing it" as we move through the book.

THE NOT-SO-*vexing* VULVA

Many of us refer to the region between our legs as our vagina, but that's not really accurate. Your vagina is internal, and the part of you that connects your outer sex parts to your uterus (and from the other opening where you pee from). The vulva is the area that you can see with a mirror, the region that features most of your lower sex parts.

I don't want to give an anatomy lecture here, but I do think it's important for your future orgasms—and all the different types you're going to be having—if we at least touch on the sexual parts of this area. In fact, this would actually be an excellent time to go grab a hand mirror or go sit in front of a mirror, spread-eagle, so you can follow along with your own.

Labia majora

That's the first thing you see. Think of this as the "case" to sex parts of you. The labia majora is essentially a set of outer lips, nicely padded, that protects the rest of the parts, but also plays a significant role in orgasms achieved via friction. It's also where the hair grows. Some say shaving this area creates more sensitivity, but that's really up to the person to whom it belongs (and also her partner, who may have a preference one way or the other). In other words, there's nothing scientific to say that shaving promotes better orgasms.

Labia minora

Tucked inside the outer labia is the part that sort of looks like a mussel. They are connected to the hood of the clitoris, which can make them quite sensitive—and also a big part of orgasms achieved via friction. They also are what provides the penis with a nice soft, wet, entry. (Lubrication does not begin in the labia minora, but this is the part of you that holds the lubrication provided by the vagina.)

Vagina

The vagina is essentially a canal—a passageway for the penis (or other object) into the woman's body. It isn't "open" all the time, like some people think. When not in use, the walls actually hold together. You can see the opening from the outside; inside it ends at the cervix, or the entrance of the uterus. It's elastic, so it can accommodate anything from a finger to birthing even a large baby, and it's lubricated. The vagina is also loaded with sensation, which we'll explore in greater depth as we get into the many kinds of orgasms there are to be enjoyed in chapter four.

quick fix } CLIT-TUTORIAL

What do you know about your clitoris? Here are some quick facts:

- A woman's height and weight do not affect the size of her clit.
- The average clitoris is roughly about a quarter of an inch in diameter "above the surface", less than an inch if you count the part that's tucked "below the surface."
- There's no effect on the size of the clitoris for women on the pill, though studies have shown that women who have given birth tend to have significantly larger clits.

- From the time a female is seven until she turns eleven, her clitoris will grow in size more than 20 percent—and then an additional 26 percent between the ages of eleven and fourteen!
- By the time a woman hits her thirties, her clitoris will have grown about four times as large as it was at the onset of puberty.
- By the time she reaches menopause, her clitoris will be about seven times the size it was at birth.

Clitoris

The clitoris has been called the "female penis," and actually, that isn't as far off the mark as it sounds. Yes, the penis is long and rodlike, but the clitoris also has a shaft, called the clitoral body, which stretches legs, called crura, kind of like the prongs on a wishbone.

Made of erectile tissue, the clitoris fills with blood when a woman is aroused and becomes engorged—which is essentially what happens to a penis when it becomes erect. Also, the clitoris is made up of thousands of nerve endings, which is what makes it something of an epicenter of female sexual stimulation. Except . . .

CLITOR-*isn't*

Okay, so now knowing what you know, that the clitoris is kind of a penis in miniature, what do you imagine to be the most important sexual organ for a woman? I know, you're thinking it must be her clitoris!

And aside from what it's made from, why wouldn't you think that the clitoris was the key to the female orgasm? It doesn't have to come from here. Read any sex manual and you can't get away from the clitoris and how only by properly nurturing this seemingly wee, little knot of nerves is the only way to ever please a woman.

Of course, there's truth in that; the problem arises when all the focus is put solely on this part. When a woman essentially becomes like a sexual target, with the clitoris as the bull's-eye, the rest of her body is ignored as a "miss." The truth of the matter is this: If a woman's body is a dartboard, then the bull's-eye is several feet off—the real target is right on top of her sexy shoulders.

> Why is orgasm the crux of losing inhibition? Studies have shown that when a woman climaxes, all the "fear" centers in her brain shut down.

BRAIN *power*!

The brain is actually the most influential sex organ for women, and for all kinds of reasons. First, we'll explore the physical.

Researchers are still hammering out exactly what role the brain plays in sexual response, and how it's different for women and men, but I will do a short overview on what they do know.

The human brain features a cool little section sometimes called a "Pleasure Center," sometimes called the "Reward Circuit," which essentially tracks everything that makes us happy. Anatomically speaking, the areas of the brain that get a charge from the pleasure center include the **amygdala**, which is in charge of regulating emotion; the **VTA (ventral tegmental area)**, which releases dopamine—the brain chemical that helps increase heart rate and blood pressure; the **cerebellum**, which is in charge of muscle function; and the **pituitary gland**, which releases so many feel-good substances into our systems, including pain-reducing beta-endorphins, trust-enhancing oxytocin, and bond-strengthening vasopressin.

So, in short, there's a system in your brain for enjoying sex and having orgasms. It's built into your blueprint, ladies. It's as much a part of your makeup as breathing. It's programmed into you just like walking. It's as natural as sneezing. You pretty much do all these things without thinking about them—so why can't orgasming be one of them?

---

quick fix } **LOSE CONTROL**

Did you know that both men and women literally "lose control" during orgasm? And that's not just being dramatic. Behind your left eye is the part of the brain called the "lateral orbitofrontal cortex," and it's the part of you that controls reason and behavior. When you have orgasm, this part of the brain actually shuts down!

Here's another neat little nugget of knowledge about orgasms and the brain. Researchers who have followed brain patterns in studies have proven that when you fake an orgasm, none of those feel-good hormones are triggered by your pleasure center. When you fake your orgasms, you're cheating your partner, and more importantly, you're cheating yourself out of so many benefits. And yet we do it all the time. This tendency has a lot to do with one's connection to their partner and is something we'll talk more about later. The brain exerts incredible control over female sexual response, both psychologically and emotionally. For the moment we are going to stick with the physical here and get more into the mental aspects in chapter 3.

quick fix } **SENSUAL SEDUCTION**

Studies have shown that the best orgasms are the ones in which all your senses are engaged. Interestingly enough, they've also found that when you're lying down, your senses are less, well, sensitive. Just another reason to explore the many sexy options outside the standard missionary position!

oh, THE NERVE!

Now we know that there is a framework in the brain actually in place for us to enjoy orgasms and all their benefits. But none of it could be possible without the incredible network of nerves that connect our brains to our many pleasure points. And such "nerve" there is: Did you know that the clitoris alone is comprised of more than eight thousand nerves? It's amazing to consider the intensity of sensation concentrated in an area about as large as a pea or the head on an eraser on a pencil.

But the clitoris isn't the only place we have all these ready-receptors, which is why we are actually able to enjoy orgasms from places other than just the standard we're used to (but we'll get into that in a bit).

The *pudendal nerve* is the one that tells our brains that fun stuff is happening around our clitoris and that the brain needs to take notice. Anatomically, while we're quite different from men down there (Of course! Of course!), the guys also have this nerve which essentially connects their penis and scrotum to their brains. So while there's that joke about "the little head and the big head," both these heads do, in fact, speak.

The **pelvic nerve** connects the brain to the rectum in both women and men, and in women, transmits messages from the cervix and vagina.

Now here's where it starts to get more interesting, and here's where I want you to really start thinking about all the possibilities for orgasm there are built right into your body. The *hypogastric nerve* runs from the brain to the uterus and cervix (to the prostate in guys). Did you even know cervical orgasms were possible? They sure are—and they're awesome.

The *vagus nerve*, which relays information from the cervix, uterus, and vagina, operates a bit differently between women and men and is actually the most intriguing of all. Why? All the nerves in the body run through the spinal cord, except this one. "So what?" you may yawn. Here's the thing. Up until recently, no one really paid that much attention to this nerve—or even that it ran through the pelvic region. Then, in a study done on women with severed spinal cords (Dr. Barry Komisaruk and Dr. Beverly Whipple of Rutgers University, 2004), it was discovered that these *paralyzed* women were able to feel stimulation of their cervixes and even have orgasms—that weren't faked because MRIs documented the brain activity. Pretty amazing, right?

Here's more: In August 2005, Suzie Heumann, founder of Tantra. com, wrote a piece for *The Huffington Post* in which she surmised that belting out your favorite song could lead to you having an orgasm—if you did it correctly. In her article entitled "What do Singing, Throats, and the Vagus Nerve Have to Do With Orgasm?" she playfully postulates that the breathing involved in powerful singing might lead to orgasm. She explains, "When we open up to sing that fully, especially songs that have a deep, lower resonance to them, we are triggering and using our vagus nerve."

Considering how amazing the vagus nerve is, we should hope that science will do more to help us learn how to harness its power! At least for now, we can take a cue from Heumann, who writes,

Opening up the mouth, chest cavity (through slow, deep breathing) and orgasmic capacities via the vagus nerve may lead to powerful orgasms and possibly multiples and female ejaculation. When women emit deep, low sounds from their abdomens and with their mouths wide open this can sometimes lead to longer lasting, powerful orgasms and even female ejaculation . . . . the vagus nerve connects all of these functions, throat, chest, cervix and uterus, and that when they are utilized to the fullest extent of the nerve, and all of its endings, the nerve becomes so activated that it produces out of body pleasure that is more than the sum of its parts, so to speak.

Makes a pretty good case for letting yourself go with the moment and have a screaming orgasm, don't you think?

ORGASMS—WHERE, WHY . . . AND HOW

Most everyone knows about the clitoral orgasm, the most common orgasm women have. But did you know there are others—many others? If there are nerves there, it can O. Check it out!

Clitoral O

The most common and obvious orgasm, the clitoral orgasm, is achieved by stimulating the clitoris—an organ in the body that has no other purpose than as a hotbutton to happiness. What could be better than that!

Vaginal O

Remember all those nerves we talked about; the walls of the vagina are loaded with them! (The first third of the vagina, starting from the entrance, has the most.)

G-Spot O

This can be a very cool and intense kind of orgasm, but a lot of women resist it because as it comes on, it feels like you're going to pee the bed and all over your partner. Relax—you aren't! It only feels that way because your G-spot is actually located close to the urethra, in the vagina, along the upper front wall. The exact location varies among women, but most G-spots are located two to three inches inside the vagina.

Cervical O

The cervix is the gateway to the uterus—and also a potential gateway to pleasure if manipulated correctly!

Breast and/or Nipple O

Some women (and men) have very sensitive nipples and breasts and have been known to O by manipulation of these parts alone.

Anal O

Like the vagina, the anus is also loaded with nerve endings, and as I have said "If it has nerves, it can O."

Sensory O

This is an orgasm you can have without having any of your sexy parts touched. Don't believe me? Well, just wait till we get to chapter 4!

NOW *you* KNOW

An orgasm is a lot more involved than just "pushing a button." It's a full-body event that affects places in you well beyond what you usually think of as being your sexy parts. Being aware of this is the first step to having more orgasms—and better ones—and to start exploring pleasure centers you never even knew you had!

Now I promised you that orgasms are good for you—really and truly physically (and psychologically) beneficial. In the next chapter, we're going to get into just how good.

CHAPTER 2

THE *MAGIC* REMEDY

"An enema under the influence of Ecstasy would probably feel much like this."
—GERMAINE GREER, JOURNALIST AND AUTHOR, ON ORGASM

There's a pretty popular saying that "love is a drug"—and people also often think that sex is just that, especially good sex. But that's definitely not where we're going here. Because there's a huge difference between what a drug does for you and what a vitamin has to offer.

Whether prescribed or recreational, a drug treats a symptom. It alters things for a limited time, and then there's a crash—and another dose is needed immediately. There may also be unwanted side effects.

Now a vitamin, on the other hand, takes a more holistic approach to a situation. You don't treat a symptom with a vitamin, you use it to help build a foundation of good health. A vitamin is essentially a supplement in a much larger system of smart choices, an important element within a larger context. A vitamin enhances. Its benefits are layered and far-reaching, not just a zapping of a targeted pain or other element.

Especially in the case of Vitamin O, it's something you can take as much as you want to take, without any worry of toxicity or buildup in your system—because Vitamin O is all about release. Add regular doses of Vitamin O to your regimen, and the results will benefit you for life.

In this chapter, we'll dive in to all the health benefits of sex and orgasm for women, and we'll show why a daily dose of Vitamin O is just what this doctor orders every time! As the proven healing and revitalizing power of sex and orgasm is revealed, we'll see without a doubt how orgasm is indeed the "magic remedy" to heal and restore us, and to build a foundation for better overall health.

> Forget echinacea. Did you know that having sex just once a week can boost your immunity by 30 percent? So imagine the benefits of getting down and dirty three, five, or even ten times a week!

O, MAGIC o

We all get rundown from time to time. We don't sleep well. We eat things we're not supposed to eat. We gain weight when there's no solid medical reason for us to be gaining weight. We all get in ruts of not really taking good enough care of ourselves. We feel like the effort to turn things around takes more energy than we are willing or able to expend. But turning the situation around is easy. There's absolutely no reason to suffering any of this when the solution is as easy as taking a daily dose of vitamins!

The power and the potency of the female orgasm has, for the most part, been buried in general studies about sex and health. Well, that's going to change right now. We're going to get to the nut of why sex and orgasms are so helpful and beneficial for women especially. By the time you get to the end of this chapter, you should be clamoring to cuddle up with your partner (or your vibrator) and get your "medicine." This chapter features the main reasons why.

---

quick fix } **FEEL THE BURN**

Sex burns calories—about 100 for an average 30-minute session. That's actually more than tennis! And when you "work out" in all the right positions, think about how successfully you can tone your tummy, thighs, and even your tush.

HORMONE *"therapy"*

Studies have proven time and again that having regular sex boosts the body's production of essential hormones like **PEA (phenylethylamine)**, which speeds the metabolism of fat. On top of that, it also curbs those killer cravings for crazy foods you know you should not be eating. It regulates your appetite so you don't feel hungry when you're not. And if you're overeating because you're bored, I'd say sex is more fun than a sandwich or sundae, any way you stack it.

Another hormone that gets released in your system when you have a good release is **DHEA (dehydroepiandrosterone)**. While researchers have been experimenting for years with this substance, it doesn't get nearly as much attention as some of the other hormones involved in sex and sexual release. So let's give it some play.

One of the main associations DHEA has is that it's purportedly an antiaging "potion." Well, production of DHEA has been noted to promote more supple skin, meaning bye, bye crow's feet! But some of the other antiaging properties have yet to be documented, for example, whether DHEA has any bearing on aging issues having to do with increased muscle strength and mass, endurance, and glucose tolerance.

DHEA is also currently being studied as a substance that possibly combats depression and eases symptoms associated with menopause.

One of the more interesting studies was done on body fat. Researchers at the Washington University School of medicine found that women who were given supplements of DHEA lost 10.2 percent of their body fat. Great! But you don't have to pop a pill to get something you can have a heck of a lot more fun making. O is the kind of vitamin that's just as beneficial to make as it is to take!

Regular sex also releases *serotonin*, a neurotransmitter that, tying in with the above, is believed to quell junk food cravings. But it's bigger than that. There's a whole wealth of studies that credit the production of serotonin with a decrease in depression—or, more like it, a lack of serotonin leads to depression. Why? As a neurotransmitter, serotonin hits various receptors that regulate emotions; when there isn't enough serotonin hitting these receptors, depression, anxiety, panic, and other unpleasant emotions result.

Anything that helps release this substance into your system is a good thing. Diet and exercise can play a role, but neither of these has a direct line to serotonin release like having an orgasm does. Antidepressants are believed also to influence serotonin levels, but these can also impede your ability to have orgasms—which we'll get into a bit later on.

What does all of this mean? Well, it looks like "being hormonal" is actually a really good thing when it comes to sex and mood—as well as your overall sense of well-being.

So we've seen how regular sex and orgasms can help make you thin, young, and happy. Now let's look at how it can make you healthy.

FIGHT *off* COLDS AND FLU

To ward off colds, we swallow huge amounts of orange juice and other fluids. We dose up on echinacea and zinc (the latter of which has been shown in recent studies to do very little if anything at all to boost our immune systems). And if, God forbid, we do get sick, we bloat ourselves with chicken soup, slurping it up like it's the last food on earth, and then stumble around like the walking dead as we drug ourselves up and dry ourselves out on anything from over the counter that promises relief. For some of us, saline becomes our best friend. And to think we could save ourselves all this grief by just allowing ourselves to have regular orgasms!

What's another benefit of Vitamin O? Studies have now uncovered that having frequent orgasms actually raises levels of the antigen *immunoglobulin* **A** in our systems, the antibody expressly responsible for fighting off colds and flu. In fact, women who engage in regular sexual activity have been found to have one-third higher levels of immunoglobulin A. What would you rather have, sex or a flu shot? Think about it!

And think about this, the other side of the coin. If you're not having regular orgasms, you're not getting the benefit and boost of these high immunoglobulin A levels. So not having orgasms—not having enough good orgasms—can actually make you sick. Another excellent reason to make sure you get your daily dose.

RUB *out* INFECTION

Two of the most common irritating pelvic ailments can be cleared up— even avoided altogether—with regular orgasms.

The bad bacteria that cause urinary tract infections (UTIs) are literally flushed out by the cervix when a woman has an orgasm. If you have an existing UTI and feel the overwhelming urge to masturbate, this is actually part of the reason why: It's your body telling you to do something about it, just like a craving in pregnancy is your body's way of telling you it needs a nutrient, like calcium, and tricks you into eating that whole pint of delicious ice cream to get it.

The other is cervical infection. Studies have shown that orgasms can ward off and even eradicate cervical infections as orgasm "tents" or opens the cervix. Like the case with a UTI. In her book *Sex: A Natural History*, Joann Ellison Rodgers explains how this process of "tenting" causes acidity in the cervical fluid to rise, which increases the number of helpful bacteria and flushes out the harmful type.

INCONTIN-*not*!

As we get older, one of the main complaints we women sometimes have is incontinence. Especially in women who have had babies, for some reason we are left to dread sneezing and laughing as never before. But guess what? Here, again, plenty of sex and regular orgasms can help! It all has to do with strengthening that pelvic floor of yours. One of the main reasons you're not able to "hold it in" like you used to is that your pelvic floor weakens over time. But you don't have to lie back and let that happen to you!

When you're at the height of orgasm, your uterus actually "lifts" off your pelvic floor, increasing pelvic muscle tension, which strengthens it and adds to your pleasure. And you can also help it along!

The next time you have sex (which should be tonight, by the way), tighten those Kegels and relax them over and over. Not only will it create a pleasurable sensation on your lover's appendage, it will strengthen the area where your orgasms happen, causing them to become stronger and more powerful—as you make that pelvic floor more powerful. (Even when you're not having sex, still do those Kegels when you can. The benefits are so worth it—especially considering how little effort they take to do. Every time it occurs to you, do twenty or thirty. You'll see the results quickly!)

FEEL GREAT *period*

Studies have also shown that women who had sex at least once a week were more likely to have more regular menstrual cycles. Also, it's been shown that regular orgasms also reduce cramps and the severity of them.

Having more orgasms means having higher levels of estrogen in your blood, which translates to a lower risk of type 2 diabetes, overall better cardiovascular health, and much less bad cholesterol in your system. (Alarmingly, there have been other studies which have proven conclusively that not having orgasms can actually have a negative impact on the cardiovascular health of women. A much more serious negative health effect than the common cold!)

When you have a better cardiovascular system, you're going to be in better shape to fight off heart disease and even some cancers. That's a scientific fact!

> In a study conducted by the AARP, it was found that for people ages fifty and over, the ones who described their level of health as excellent or very good were the ones having sex at least once a week!

SLEEP MORE *soundly*

Here's one of those "vicious cycle" situations. When you are overtired, your libido is lessened, which means you don't want sex. And if you're fatigued and overtired, due to lack of sleep, you especially don't. Except that sex and orgasm do actually promote sleep. Which means the thing you want least is what's going to help you the most.

Are orgasms good for sleeping? Of course. Sex exerts energy, and the more into it you are, the more energy you're going to expend. But "sex-ercise" aside, orgasms themselves are a natural tranquilizer. They relieve tension, which is huge in helping us get to sleep and stay asleep. As our heart beats faster, the increased blood flow rushes all that good stuff we talked about around in our systems. The relaxing of the muscle tautness that increases as we anticipate release helps relieve all those nasty, annoying tensions you trap in your nervous system over the course of a day.

After orgasm, in women, the blood pressure starts to gradually decrease, promoting relaxation, along with the calming, soothing release of all those wonderful endorphins. If you've had a particularly stressful day, why drag all that drama to bed with you when you and your partner can work it out together—or just yourself!

And if you're feeling too tired to have sex—maybe it's time to break that vicious cycle once and for all.

HAPPY BODY, HAPPY MIND— AND HAPPY *spirit*

Remember our friend DHEA? One of the other amazing attributes DHEA has is that it has been shown to improve brain function. Studies have demonstrated that people with higher levels of DHEA do better on tests while those with lower levels don't score as well. Other tests are currently being performed to test DHEA levels and occurrences of Alzheimer's, and most are concluding that people with higher levels of DHEA are less likely to be afflicted by Alzheimer's than those with lower levels. Talk about a long-term plan! An orgasm a day keeps dementia away?

In addition to improving your cranial capacity, having regular orgasms has also been shown to boost self-esteem. In a study conducted by the University of Texas, published in the *Archives of Sexual Behavior*, "boosting self-esteem" was one of the main reasons people have sex. And Cambridge-based sex, marriage, and family therapist Gina Ogden confirmed in an article on WebMD that "one of the reasons people say they have sex is to feel good about themselves. Great sex begins with self-esteem, and it raises it. If the sex is loving, connected, and what you want, it raises it." Whether it's through self-pleasuring or pleasuring yourself through a partner, exploring, understanding, and articulating what satisfies you sexually is actually a giant boost to your self-esteem.

Think about it. Knowing what you want, going after it, and getting it—what makes you feel better about yourself than that?

And, something most everyone already knows: Sex and orgasms help relieve stress. Whether with your partner or by yourself, taking a break from the emotionally taxing aspects of your life, like managing your job and family and finances, and finding a quiet place to focus on yourself or on each other for just a small slice of a day will help ease the aggravation of everything else that's been eating away at you. And when we become sexually aroused, our levels of dopamine and adrenaline become elevated, which means we get happier.

On a spiritual level, just take a look at the ancients. They saw sex as something sacred and uplifting and saw orgasm as a conduit for connection to ourselves and the energy of the universe. There's a lot to be said about the spiritual aspect of sex, I could write a book on that alone. But we'll touch on it briefly in chapter 4 when we discover the "Spiritual O."

Yep. Regular orgasms will make you feel good while you're having them, and they are indeed the gift that keeps giving.

> Studies have proven again and again that people who report having good sex lives also report a better quality of life overall.

THE OTHER MAGIC *o*

While this is all great stuff, I'd say the icing on the cake definitely has to be that Vitamin O releases the other Magic O: oxytocin. Known as the body's "cuddle hormone," oxytocin is the body's feel-good hormone and reigns supreme on the list of good stuff, as it alone can actually do what each hormone we talked about already does—and more.

Here's one biggie we haven't really gotten into yet with the others: pain management. Do you have a headache (and not the one you're pretending to have because you don't feel like having sex—though this will cure that one too)? Oxytocin released into our systems helps us manage pain. So using back pain, bad knees, or any other physical ailment that causes you pain or discomfort as an excuse not to have sex is actually counterintuitive. What would be much more effective, on so many levels, is for you to just lie there and let your lover bestow all kinds of lascivious love treats on you—a much better bargain than choking down a pricey pill for the pain relief you need!

There's another big plus when it comes to lots of oxytocin running through our bodies: High oxytocin levels make us want to connect to others. So the more we share orgasms with our partners, the more we want to share orgasms with them. Yep. Thanks to the other O, frequent, powerful orgasms actually improve our bond with our partners!

quick fix } CAREER CHANGER

All the physical benefits you can get from having an orgasm a day should be enough—but did you know it can also help you advance in your career? A team of Scottish researchers recently discovered that people have an easier time speaking in public after a sexual release. Considering that the number one fear people have (more so than death) is public speaking, the argument can truly be made that orgasms are life-savers!

NOW *you* KNOW

One of the greatest tonics a woman can take to seal in her good health costs nothing, can be achieved with or without company, and has benefits well beyond the initial pleasure it provides.With this knowledge, you should be wanting and working at having at least one orgasm every day.

But can you believe only 30 percent of women always have an orgasm while 45 percent guess they have them "most of the time"? Nearly 75 percent of women don't climax during intercourse, and as many as 50 percent admit to being mostly dissatisfied with the way they have orgasms and the kinds they have. But here's the most shocking stat of all: As many as 10 to 15 percent of women say they've *never had an orgasm*. What? WHAT?! When you consider that the percentage of men that haven't ever had an orgasm—that would be zero percent—why are women missing out?

In the next chapter, we'll look at the main reasons women are not getting the O they need and deserve, and we'll pose some solutions to overcome all the bullshit that's blocking the bliss.

CHAPTER 3

THE
secret
INGREDIENT

"I may not be a great actress but I've become the greatest at screen orgasms. Ten seconds of heavy breathing, roll your head from side to side, simulate a slight asthma attack and die a little."
—CANDICE BERGEN

I f you are an actor and you are being offered a pile of money to pretend you're getting off in front of the camera, faking an orgasm is a good idea. Otherwise—not a chance. Not with all we discovered in the last chapter about how amazingly good they are for you!

So why does it happen? Why do so many women not have orgasms—or not have sex for that matter?

Sometimes there are medical reasons women have difficulty climaxing, and we'll touch on that only slightly in this book; my area of expertise has to do more with the emotional and sexological end of the spectrum. And believe it or not, an astounding 90 percent of a woman's orgasm problems have to do with what goes on in her head. Anxiety, inhibition, and sometimes even ignorance all play a role, but there's also her ideas on what she should expect, as well as how she imagines he thinks she should be acting. Number of men this holds true for: zero.

And that's not the worst of it. It actually puts in motion a pretty vicious cycle. When a woman has difficulty climaxing, she gets frustrated and turns off even trying to have orgasms. Then, because of that, she might start turning off sex altogether. In addition to being absolutely terrible for her, this also now creates a terrible situation with her partner, who, as a result of her lack of interest in sex, becomes frustrated and confused. Why doesn't his lover want to have sex with him? Is it something he did or didn't do? Is he not doing it right? Will she ever want to have sex again? And, at the very worst, should he be looking someplace else to get it?

At this point, it's no longer just a matter of your own physical and mental health; now it has to do with the physical and mental health of your partner and also your relationship. Not having sex puts a real strain on a relationship. Remember that sex is like glue for a couple: Take away that connection and it's possible, even likely, that the relationship can fall apart.

But it never has to get to that point—not with good communication, which is the true secret ingredient to having orgasms and better orgasms, which we'll demonstrate time and again as we move through the second section of this book. For the purposes of this chapter now, we'll look into the reasons why women don't have orgasms and find solutions for getting over not having orgasms. What it takes, essentially, is seeing that there's an issue and working together to overcome it. Because in many cases, sometimes what sparks the inability for a woman not to be able to have an orgasm is that she and her partner are not connecting as well as they could. Talk about a vicious cycle!

In this chapter, I'll explain some of the reasons women don't orgasm, whether that means they're unable to orgasm or they just need an easier method. I'll introduce you to some of my clients (names changed, of course), who have struggled with sexual dysfunction issues and not being able to climax, and show how I helped them. I'll also offer solutions to getting over what's holding you back and bringing that libido back!

> Do you know your emotional IQ? Studies have shown that women with high emotional intelligence have more frequent and intense orgasms.

NO *O*? O NO!

In the last chapter, we discovered that an alarming number of women either don't have orgasms or even an interest in sex "anymore" or believe they've never had an orgasm. Now it's time to figure out why.

A woman who has never had an orgasm before is known as "preorgasmic." Interestingly enough, the term used to be anorgasmic, which, like the term asexual means "without." Thankfully, the new term is *hopeful*—it means you haven't had an orgasm before, but you aren't "without" the ability to have one; you simply haven't discovered how yet. Lucky for you, this book is packed with all kinds of wonderful methods to try. The term preorgasmic is mainly used for younger women, under the age of twenty, but a woman can be preorgasmic at any age.

Now, if you're "post-orgasmic" (okay, not the scientific term but it makes sense in this context), meaning you've had orgasms in your life and you can't seem to get back there, the rest of this chapter is really for *you*. Not being able to have an orgasm for a woman can be a frustrating and even sometimes debilitating thing, but the good news is it's also a situation that can be fixed once you get to the heart of the matter. As we move through this chapter, I'll show you how I helped others get their sex life—and, as a result, their relationships—back on track.

THE MISSING *o*

Gail, a married mother of two, came to see me with her husband, Dirk. After a difficult couple of years, she finally admitted to him that she rarely, if ever, had orgasms when she was intimate with him, and that this had been going on for some time. Gail had chosen to ignore the situation, hoping it would resolve itself, choosing to instead pretend that everything was okay so as to spare Dirk's feelings, but also not wanting to face that there was something wrong with her. "Except what seemed to hurt Dirk more was not that I hadn't been able to climax with him, but hadn't been able to share that I hadn't with him," she told me.

Gail and Dirk had been married five years, together another two before that. Over the course of their relationship, they both remembered times when the sex was great and other times it had tapered off. What was worrying them now was that the "off" periods had never been so long before—and what if they were never going to turn around to "on" again?

After meeting with them both together and separately, Gail was finally able to voice one of the issues she was having. "I don't like it when Dirk asks me after sex or sometimes during 'Did you have an orgasm?' It makes me feel so pressured, you know, like if I'm not getting off, he's not going to either, and we're just wasting our time. Worse than that is when he decides he'd like for us to come together. It's been hard enough trying to get there on a separate timeline—but the same one? That just seems impossible to me! I guess it's just easier to fake it, to take the pressure off. Except now it seems like I can't break the habit. I don't really know what to do."

The problem with Gail wasn't unusual, and I assured her that it wasn't. Because we don't necessarily orgasm as quickly and effortlessly as our partners, all women at some time or another in their lives have faked Os because they feel it's too much pressure to have them. Unfortunately, it creates another one of those vicious cycles. If you take the pressure off yourself, you will actually orgasm more easily, and that's how I advised her. I also told her that she shouldn't feel embarrassed or meek to tell Dirk that whatever he may be doing might not be working, in a gentle way. Because by faking orgasm, what she's doing is pretty much letting Dirk know that what he's doing is working, which cheats them both.

"I understand your point," she told me. "But I'm really not sure how to communicate this with him. He has a tendency to be sensitive about things, and I'm worried if I tell him, he'll lose his confidence and stop enjoying sex as well."

I reminded her that sex was meant to make both partners happy and everyone involved should be enjoying themselves—that it was a team effort—and I told her how I would proceed in her shoes.

He was already aware of the problem, but I advised her to read-dress it with him. To sit him down, outside the bedroom, and explain the situation—that she had been faking orgasms because she had been finding it difficult to orgasm. I then advised her to be truthful about the situation and her feelings, to let Dirk know that when he asked her if she'd had an orgasm, it caused her to panic, which is why she'd lie and just fake it to get it over with.

Once she had explained everything in a loving, reassuring way, I told her to reinforce the fact that she had to tell him what was going on because she wanted to get back to having orgasms and to also ask that he please not ask her anymore if she's had an orgasm when they were intimate—to just rely on her to tell him when she's had one. I also let her know that he was probably going to have some questions for her, which could the following include:

- How long has this been going on?
- Why have you been lying to me?
- Have I ever satisfied you?
- Do you like having sex with me?
- What am I doing wrong?

I advised her to answer his questions honestly and directly and to be kind, loving, and reassuring when she did.

TALK THE *talk*, WALK THE *walk*

Gail and Dirk had their much-needed talk, and while Dirk was, as Gail had predicted, sensitive at first, internalizing the problem and thinking it was all his fault, what came out of the conversation was now an open window into how the two had had a longstanding communication break-down, which had actually affected other areas of their lives together, and which they were now on their way to resolving.

The heart of the matter was simple. In all the years they had been together, Gail had never expressed to Dirk *how* she enjoyed being made love to—she had pretty much just left it up to him to figure out. And because she never let him know otherwise, he thought he pretty much had it all figured out. Except that she needed more foreplay—lots of more foreplay.

Later, Gail and Dirk came back to me for advice on how to cover the bases. Following is a list of questions I created for them to help get them back on track in their situation. The objective was for Gail to look at the questions, think about the answers, and then communicate these to Dirk. If you need a tool to help you communicate your sexual needs with your partner, this list of questions can help you too:

- Do you like foreplay?
- And if so, what type do you like best?
- How long do you like foreplay to last?
- Do you reach orgasm via oral pleasure? Manual stimulation?
- Are you G-spot sensitive?
- Can you bring yourself to orgasm via self-pleasuring? How long does it take you?
- Do you have a special way of bringing yourself to orgasm—and special tricks you employ, like pressure and friction?
- Can you show your partner how to bring you to orgasm?
- Are you able to reach orgasm during sexual intercourse?
- What positions do you find easier to orgasm in?

Like Dirk, some men think that their partner's inability to have an orgasm is related to their style of making love and that can make them feel inadequate—although in some cases this is true, it can also be a personal matter for her as well as lack of communication. So instead of focusing on what your partner is doing *wrong*, focus on what you can make right. In other words, really pay attention to what makes you happy sexually and encourage your partner to keep repeating those things you want to see happen by really reinforcing the behavior when you like it. When he touches you in a way you like, moan louder, reorient your body to meet his touch, or simply say, "I love that. That feels great. Keep doing more of that!"

Remember that when it comes to sex with a long-term partner, the desire part of sex is always going to wax and wane. There are stages and phases to a love life. First comes attraction, romantic love, passion, and sex, and over time, love develops into realistic love and sex—and especially after you have kids, you need to get realistic about sex! We'll talk more about that in a bit, but just rest assured that having kids does not mean not having sex. You can still have a great sex life when you have kids—you just have to be realistic about expectations. Wherever you are in your relationship, keep in mind that sex drive is an ongoing project.

DANCE OF *desire*

Jeanine, a thirty-five-year-old photographer, came to see me recently. She considered herself happily married—except for the sex part, that is. Between the sheets, Todd apparently wasn't scoring as high as he was in other areas of being a husband.

"I have a great husband in many ways," Jeanine told me, "but in the sack he is terribly unskilled. It seems like I never orgasm with him, and I can't help but blame him over this. Instead of being fulfilled and happy after sex, I'm just plain frustrated, and my annoyance with him is starting to seep into other areas of my life. I'm worried my marriage is going to be in trouble over this."

I had the same sense that her marriage would be, if it was not already, suffering, and I asked her to be more specific with me about what wasn't working behind the bedroom door. "I've had other lovers," she confessed, "and with them, sex always felt so fluid. Like a dance. Like a dance both my other partners and I were in step with. Not to be mean, but Todd 'dances' with two left feet—not to mention that he's kind of also 'all thumbs.' Sex feels so clumsy with him, and worse than me being annoyed about it, I sometimes just lie there, well," she hedged, "bored."

I felt badly for Jeanine, and also for Todd. Maybe they weren't compatible. Maybe they should consider a trial separation to figure things out, which I suggested to her. "Oh no," Jeanine said, impassioned. "I love my husband very much, please don't get me wrong. He's such a great catch in so many other ways. I just don't understand with all the other great stuff he has going on in his life and in our relationship, why in this particular way he's kind of a dud."

I first told Jeanine that I don't believe in blaming your partner if the sex life you're sharing isn't exciting, and you can't blame somebody for your inability to orgasm. It's not their fault. As the old saying goes, "It takes two to tango." If you're not speaking up and telling your partner what works and what doesn't, you're falling down on fulfilling your end of the bargain. I urged her to tell Frank what she needed, to lead the dance for a while to get them back in step. Because sex really is a lot like dancing. One person might be more skilled or experienced than the other, but with some great communication and practice, you can work it like pros. Firm up that connection, and great sex will result.

In my experience, most of the time not being able to orgasm has to do with communication and connections—or lack of connection between a woman and her partner, and between her and her own sexuality. So the secret ingredient is as basic as "connection"—but to oneself, to one's own needs, to expressing these needs with one's partner is where it can get somewhat complicated. Now, I want to talk about the elements that take place far away from the bed that effect sex and sexual performance.

What goes on behind the bedroom door is not all that factors in to a disconnect with couples and sex. Outside factors, even the most minute and mundane of them, can affect our sexual desire. Part of the problem here is when the responsibility for these tasks seems imbalanced. Resentment and anger can kill sex drive as much as anything else. It's important to sort these things out because what can result is what we discussed earlier: that vicious cycle that starts when one party shuts down and doesn't properly communicate why.

THE PREGNANCY *paradox*

As I will explain more a bit later, pregnancy does many strange things to a woman—body, mind, and soul. Did you know that when pregnant, a woman has more hormones coursing through her body than at any other point in her life? There's no reason to believe your sex drive will be the same when you're pregnant—nor should you believe that the ease (or lack of ease) you have when you're pregnant will be consistent with other times in your life.

Take my client Alex, for instance, a twenty-nine-year-old real estate broker. She contacted me through my radio show when she was six months pregnant with her first child. She and her husband, Steve, had always had great sex. "But since I've been showing," she said, "it feels like it takes me forever to have an orgasm. Sometimes I can't have one at all, but I want to have sex all the time, even when my husband doesn't. Is this normal?"

As I said above, pregnancy and sex are a tricky combination. I told her, "Some women experience the best sex of their lives while pregnant, others have difficulty. You say that it's really been since you've been showing that you've had issues with orgasming. Is it possible you may be having inhibitions because your body is not in its normal shape?"

She agreed this could be part of the issue and also realized that it had more to it than that. "You know," she said, "I've always had the best orgasms on my back—but it's just not that comfortable lying straight on my back for long enough to have an orgasm anymore."

I agreed with her. It's true that the larger you get, the fewer options you have for positions. I recommended she try a few variations and see what happens. I did also suggest that she may, even if she isn't aware of it, be feeling insecure on some level because not all her sex initiations are met with the kind of enthusiasm with which she delivers them. "It could be that you're feeling rushed to have an orgasm because your husband doesn't seem to want sex as frequently as you do," I suggested.

It's actually very common for pregnant women to become "horn dogs" and want sex all the time. Sometimes the husbands just can't keep up! The only way I ever "got enough" during pregnancy is when I would supplement my sex life with a vibrator. Try it. You might find that a vibrator fulfills your needs and takes the pressure off—and in more ways than one.

oh BABY . . .

So first comes love, then comes marriage. And throughout this exciting time, it's all passion, fire, pleasure, and sex, sex, sex!

And then comes baby and your whole life changes—as well as your perspective on life. If whose turn to initiate sex was the focus of your relationship before, now it's whose turn is it to change diapers and give feedings and get out of bed in the middle of the night. Gone are the delicious all-night sex marathons, the sensual showers you snuck into in the wee hours just because you had the urge. And in their place, marathon walks up and down the hall to put the baby back to sleep and running the shower in the middle of the night to clear up the croup.

In the midst of all this mayhem, who has time to think about sex—and who has the inclination to have it (when, all things considered, that's just how you ended up "in this mess" to begin with)?

Amy, a forty-one-year-old stay-at-home mother, also found another unexpected letdown sexually after her daughter was born. "I came so easily when I was pregnant," she explained to me. "So why am I having a hard time now?"

I took a deep breath and explained to her that there were many, many reasons this was the case at this point in her life, but with all she had going on juggling all her new responsibilities, I decided to take it a step at a time.

I told her that there was a good, solid physiological reason she had an easier time orgasming when she was pregnant, and this seemed to relax her. "I was worried there might be something, you know, 'off' about me—in my head," she laughed. (And we'll address some of those worries here a bit later.)

I explained to her that during pregnancy, orgasms are usually different. Never mind all the hormones coursing through you at once, but when pregnant, many women have increased fluids in their clitoral and vaginal region, which makes them more orgasmic. Women who have never orgasmed might experience their first O during this time; women who have orgasmed before might even become multiorgasmic! (Just as a side note, in case you're wondering, your fetus is not in danger or in any pain or discomfort of any kind when you orgasm while pregnant. In fact, just the opposite is true. Not only does the fetus benefit from the surge of happy hormones released in you, the light contractions of the uterus also create a pleasant "rocking" for your little one. Yet another benefit of Vitamin O!)

After pregnancy, it does take your body some time to adjust to its normal hormonal levels, so it's quite common to not orgasm as easily or powerfully. "Don't worry," I assured her. "If you were able to orgasm before, you'll get it back. It just takes time."

"Time," she laughed. "I don't seem to have much of that anymore." Then she got more serious. "And I don't seem to have much sex drive anymore. I'm sure it has something to do with the difference in orgasming between then and now, but could it be more than that?"

"Well, yes, it could be," I told her, "and we'll get into that a little more as we move through this chapter. But, as I explained to Amy, her lack of sex drive probably had a lot less to do with her health and the state of her body, and her direct feelings for her husband, than she was guessing they did.

There are many factors that affect sex drive once a baby comes into your life. There are lots of physiological reasons your body and mind are in no rush to bring sexy back so quickly after childbirth. On top of the exhaustion felt from being insanely sleep-deprived, there's the healing process. Natural it may be, but giving birth to a baby is like giving birth to a train: your nether regions are wrecked and for a while. Aside from any tearing you may have experienced, or sometimes worse, the dreaded episiotomy, birth does affect your pelvic nerves and muscles, and also your vagina. Sometimes damage is done down there, even temporarily, that can make the sensual parts of you less sensitive.

If you're breastfeeding, there are many benefits for you and baby both, but sexually, there are some drawbacks. Aside from you now primarily thinking of your breasts as a food source and not a pleasure source (especially in the beginning when nursing sometimes really hurts!), breastfeeding lowers your body's levels of estradiol. And if you're wondering what that is, estradiol is the hormone that keeps you "wet" down there. So when you do feel up to resuming your sex life and you've gotten the green light from your doctor, there may be some pain and discomfort—but that can be easily remedied with a little bit of lube. Then there's the increased secretion of prolactin, which actually lowers testosterone, curbing sexual desire. Later in life, during menopause, estradiol production is reduced and testosterone levels can drop by half. This may also lead to diminished sex drive and decreased sensitivity in the erogenous zones , which can make orgasming difficult and frustrating.

So while you will do anything for your sweet little bundle of love, remember that you also love your partner. I know that with all the nearly constant responsibility, the incessant demands being made of you, and not to mention, the hell your body went to once you passed the placenta, it might be hard to see that person as anything more than another set of arms to hold the baby. Totally normal, but you have to start seeing that person as a luscious sex object again. Your health, your sanity, and your relationship actually depend on it. We'll give plenty of "hows" a little bit later in the "hands on" section.

snapping BACK

Like Amy, Shawna had issues with her sex drive after having her kids, now age two and five. For Shawna, the situation was purely physical, at least in her perception of it, which ended up affecting her emotionally. "After giving birth vaginally to two babies, both nine-pounders," she explained, "I feel a little loose down there. I don't feel like I'm really satisfying my husband anymore."

"Has he told you that?" I asked her.

"Oh no," she said. "He never says anything about it. I just feel like that's the way it is, and he won't say anything about it because he doesn't want to hurt my feelings."

We talked for a while about communication and how it's key, and how she could be feeling something that isn't necessarily true. She agreed to have a talk with him about it, but she still seemed on the fence. "I have to admit it," she hedged. "I just don't feel the same. I also rarely, if ever, have orgasms anymore. Can having kids affect my ability to have orgasms?"

This is kind of a double-edged issue. The answer here is actually both "no" and "yes." It's a tricky question because having kids means less time for sex, which naturally means fewer orgasms. But I assured her. "As far as your ability to have orgasms goes, if you had them before there is no reason you can't have them again. It might take some time to get back on track hormonally and perhaps with your body image," I said, "but if you put some effort into it, you should be fine."

"Well, I guess I can try," she said. "But what about the 'loose' issue. What if my husband says there is a difference?"

"Is he still trying to have sex with you?" I asked.

"Yes."

"Well then, if he notices at all, it probably doesn't bother him."

"But it bothers me," she said. So I talked her through some of the ways she could get her elasticity back.

I assured her that her fears were grounded and her feelings justified. It's actually quite common for women to worry that their vaginas have become too lose and wonder how they can be tightened. Whether by childbirth or other situations, when a woman feels her vagina is too loose, it can affect her self-esteem. I generally recommend Kegel exercises, which are an effective surgery-free option.

Kegel Exercises

As we discussed briefly in the last chapter, Kegel exercises are your friend for so many reasons. For one, they strengthen the pelvic floor muscles, which not only means you don't pee when you laugh or sneeze, but you also have more intense orgasms. But they're also easy, require no extra equipment, and can be done anywhere at any time—and no one will ever know (that is, unless you're *en flagrante* with your partner because this is something he will totally feel!). Here are the steps:

1. *Find the muscles.* Again, easy. The next time you pee, stop the stream. How do you do this? By tightening. What you're tightening are those muscles—see? Now you know where they are.
2. *Squeeze them.* Repeatedly. Tighten the muscles and hold for about 10 seconds (which you can increase as you go).
3. *Release and repeat.* Try it five times at first, then as many as fifty times the stronger you get.

Do these exercises a few times a day and your pelvic floor will spring back into shape in a matter of weeks.

Surgery

You can elect to have your vagina tightened through surgery, a procedure called vaginoplasty, but it is costly (it generally isn't covered by insurance), can be painful, and requires a recovery of three to sometimes six weeks, during which time you can't have sex.

In this procedure, the walls of the vaginal canal are essentially reconstructed. It's also the procedure transgendered males undergo to become female. The end product is supposed to be a smaller more toned vagina, but the big risk is that a woman sometimes has a lack of sensation in her vagina afterward. Other surgeries designed to "correct" the havoc brought on by childbirth include labioplasty, plastic surgery involving the folds of tissue on the labia, and vaginal rejuvenation, which is a nonreconstructive procedure that removes excess tissue in the vagina and tightens the walls.

So was it necessary for Shawna to consider taking such a drastic step in correcting the situation down below? No. Her husband assured her that there was no change in sensation for him, which relaxed her. But she also did the Kegels, which were not only fun when she did them while intimate with him, but also improved some problems she was having with incontinence.

life's MESSES AND STRESSES

A new baby isn't the only thing in married or coupled life that can come between you and your orgasms. Let's face it: Life is filled with buzz-killing landmines primed and ready to sabotage your libido. You have to keep an eye out for them and try to step around them. From the demands your job can put on you to being pulled in seventeen different directions each and every day as you carpool your kids and their friends to various activities and events, there aren't many occasions in daily life to feel sexy. That's why you have to take them—you have to be able to see past what you have to endure each day and turn your focus instead on how you can reward yourself and your partner for getting through it.

Instead of dwelling on how strapped you are for time and energy, think instead of how nice it will be to reconnect with your partner or yourself once the tasks are behind you, and treat yourselves to an orgasm or two—or more! Why not? Keeping in optimum physical and mental health helps manage your stress. Too much stress can kill you, but first it kills your sex life.

BRINGING IT BACK TO *you*

When you take time for yourself, even just twenty minutes a day, focusing on yourself and not on grocery lists, bills, or after-school activities, you'll be taking an important step to come back to the sexual you. I'm not saying you need to spend this "you" time on sexual pursuits—though of course you can, if that means sneaking away with an erotic book is what makes you happy. It just has to be something that's purely, selfishly (in a good way) about you. It could be a walk or a jog, a dance class, a pedicure, and if you can manage to get away for longer sometimes, all the better: a movie, a quiet dinner out with the characters in a novel you're reading, anything you can think of that will give you pleasure and that you share with only one person. Yourself.

If what you decide you'd like to do involves exercise, all the better! Exercise releases all those wonderful endorphins into your system. Cardio gets your heat racing; flexibility and strength training make you limber and give you stamina—all great for sex! And doing squats and lunges will also increase your blood flow to your pelvic region.

Yoga and Pilates are especially good "sexercises." In addition to strengthening your core, they also strengthen your pelvic muscles and floor, which all help you to have orgasms. In yoga, your mind is also part of the exercising, as you consciously release all the bad, negative energy from you with each pose and change in position.

Exercise can improve orgasms, but can you have an orgasm during exercise? You sure can! A Yo-gasm after or during yoga; a Pi-Gasm after or during Pilates.

quick fix } **MEDITATE ON IT**

Another great way to reconnect with yourself? Try meditation. Not only will it give you a time-out for yourself, studies have shown that practicing meditation has improved arousal in women and helped them achieve better orgasms!

serious BONDAGE

Just as you need to take time for yourself to get you refocused on sex, so should you take time with your partner, to refocus on your relationship and reconnect. It could be as simple as waking up a little earlier in the morning to share a quiet cup of coffee before the kids get up and the craziness begins.

In this time, make an effort to talk—to really communicate— about what you might be feeling. If the chores load doesn't feel balanced, see if a solution can be found. Once you can communicate comfortably and openly on that level, it will be easier to express your needs sexually.

Here are some quick and easy ways to reconnect. They'll take only seconds but the impact can last a lifetime:

- Make your hellos and goodbyes more passionate by kissing for thirty seconds or more when you do.

- Take any opportunity you can to touch your partner, by holding hands, placing your hand on the arm of the person you love when you speak to them, hug, and snuggle whenever possible.
- Take baths and showers together.
- Help your partner get dressed in the morning.
- Tuck your partner into bed at night.
- Go for walks together.
- Do chores together so it goes faster.
- Speak to your partner with loving, kind words regularly.
- Date at least once a week—either going out to dinner or taking an occasional day date, spending at least an hour alone together.
- Turn the mundane into an opportunity to connect by running errands together.

These are just a few suggestions. Now what can you think of?

OUT WITH THE *old* . . .

Bonding is important for long-term couples; it's also essential for new ones. When you start a new relationship, you're still sometimes "bound" to the way things had been with your former partner, and it doesn't always matter how much time has passed between partners. When you have a regular partner, you get programmed into their patterns. When you have a new partner, sometimes the sex doesn't seem to be working because you're still programmed a certain way and need to reboot.

For example, Alison, a forty-two-year-old divorced banker, called in to one of my radio shows worried that while she cared deeply for her new boyfriend, things might not work out because of the sex.

"I used to have orgasms so easily with my last partner during oral," she explained, "and now I don't with my new partner. What's going on?"

She needed to be deprogrammed. I told her, "It's more than likely that what's affecting your ability to orgasm here is your comfort level with your new partner—not their skills or lack of skills. There is an adjustment period that you go through with every new partner. If you are not happy with the way your partner is orally pleasing you, then you need more time adjusting to them, and if you don't like what they are doing to you orally, then you need to speak up. If your last partner did it better, teach your new partner how to satisfy you without bringing up your last partner, of course!"

quick fix } HOW TO DEPROGRAM YOURSELF FROM AN EX-LOVER: A FEW SIMPLE STEPS

- *Hold back.* Don't jump right in to a new relationship. After a breakup, give yourself time to heal before taking the plunge again. Otherwise, what you may be doing on some level is not looking for a new partner at all, but a replacement for the one you lost.
- *Focus on yourself.* After a breakup, it's easy to feel lost when all you feel is loss. Why not change that focus? Instead of worrying about what you no longer have, think of all the things you can have—passions and dreams and other things inside you that may have been neglected when you focused so much of yourself on your last partner.
- *Meditate.* Detox yourself from the past by taking some time to do some relaxing, reflective meditative exercises.

> • *Learn to enjoy your own company.* Only when you can make yourself a complete person on your own are you ready to share yourself with someone else.

There's a learning curve with a new partner, just as there is with any new experience. Bend with it, and use it. When your new partner does something that feels great, let him know with your words or your moans. And if you want something specific, tell him "I really like it when you use your tongue like that," and so forth. Be sure to reinforce the pleasurable behavior by saying "I really like it when . . . " And then when you reach orgasm, let him know how it happened.

Take these steps, talk it through. You will both feel really good about the whole experience, and you might be amazed at how much better the sex will get.

other FACTORS

Having too much stress in your life and not communicating in a relationship are some of the reasons sex can suffer and reaching orgasm can be difficult, but on top of these more emotionally focused factors are the physical factors. Libido can be as much about what's going on with your body as it is with your mind, so as you work with your partner to address what may be hindering your desire.

lube JOB

Vaginal dryness is one of the easiest issues to address. If a lack of lubrication is the issue getting in the way of you enjoying sex and wanting to have it often, there are so many options on the market, over the counter and even prescription. You don't have to go into an adult store to find them either (though if that's the kind of excursion you and your lover can take, that can really get you going!).

Whether you have an issue with dryness or not, having plenty of lube at the ready can make sex a lot more fun—and a lot more pleasant when your natural vaginal secretions sometimes aren't enough. Here's a breakdown of some of the types of lubes on the market these days.

Water-Based

I myself prefer water-based lubes as they are the least likely to stain your sheets or intimate apparel, are less likely to cause irritation, and are compatible to use with condoms. They're also much easier to clean off your body and your toys—just a little warm water and soap and you're done! Water-based lubes are also less expensive than some of the other varieties. And some do come in flavors, if you're into that kind of thing! Just be careful: If you have sensitive skin, these may cause irritation. Best to try them out a little bit at a time!

One of the most common water-based lubes is KY jelly, which is thicker than water and also a bit sticky. They now make different varieties of KY—some that are not as thick, some that actually warm when contact is made with the skin. Astroglide is actually thinner and lasts longer than KY, but it's also more expensive. Again, it really comes down to what's important to you.

The downside of water-based lubes is that they do dry a bit more quickly than the other types, and some people find the sticky factor, well, icky.

Petroleum-Based

Petroleum-based lubes, such as Vaseline, are thick and delightfully slippery, but they are not without risk. Because they tend to erode latex and rubber, they are not recommended to use with latex condoms, dia-phragms, cervical caps, and even some sex toys. They are excellent, how-ever, when it comes to sexually massaging the penis or the clitoris (they are not for use inside the vagina as they can cause irritation).

Mineral Oil

Also thick and satisfying, mineral oil, because of the very nature of what it is (i.e., oil), is a great choice for lubing up in the shower or bathtub or other wet—and wild as you make them—venues. It's also available on the shelves at the drugstore so it's easy to get. While it's not strictly forbidden for vaginal use, some people do complain about irritation when it's used internally. As always, proceed with caution, and a little bit at a time.

Silicone-Based

These are popular because they are very thin and they last a long time. Also, you don't need much more than a drop to get great results. On the downside, because they're fairly new on the market, they tend to be more expensive and also hard to find. They're safe with most sex toys (though not ones made from silicone), and latex and rubber get the green light. If you can't find these in your local drugstore, try the Internet. Two of the best and most widely available are Eros and ID Millennium.

Natural Oils

This is just what you think it is: edible oils in your pantry, like olive oil and vegetable oil. While these oils are very easy to come by (no pun intended), innocently stocked and shelved in your local grocery store, they are not great to use with latex or rubber because they are known to damage these materials. In the plus column, they are safer for vaginal use than some of the other options available and, if not imported, are quite inexpensive.

quick fix } **MY *FAVORITE* LUBES**

- *Water-based*: Astroglide, KY, Pjur, Slippery Stuff Gel, Juntos, Wet Naturals, Intimate Organics Hydra, Sliquid H2O
- *Flavored*: System Jo H2O, ID Juicy Lubes
- *Silicone*: Eros, Wet Platinum, Pink. (By the way, KY and Astroglide also make great silicone lubes.)
- *Anal*: Sliquid Sassy Booty Lube (we'll talk more about anal lubes in later chapters, but you have to admit this is a great name for this product!)

WHEN DRYNESS *isn't* THE ISSUE

There are many devices available to enhance sex when simple lube is not the issue. One device, called the Estring, is a vaginal ring that does just that. There are also vaginal pumps available on the market which are designed to pump more blood into the labia and clitoris and can increase sensitivity in that region, making it easier to orgasm.

With any of these products or devices, be sure to always follow the directions and don't overuse them. Also, speak with your doctor to see if they're right for you.

A new product out there that I like a lot is called the NuGyn Eros Therapy Device. This small handheld gadget is FDA approved and proven to assist women specifically with arousal and orgasmic disorders. It works as a gentle vacuum that increases blood flow to the clitoris and pelvic region, which not only increase sensitivity and therefore the likelihood of orgasm, but also enhances vaginal lubrication. You have to talk to your doctor about this device as it's available by prescription only—and be sure to follow the directions!

(Think Viagra is a guy thing? Think again! Researchers testing the little blue pill have found that Viagra improved sexual response in 72 percent of women they tested.)

TEST(OSTERONE) IT *out*

You may associate testosterone with men, but it's the hormone in both men and women most essential to sexual desire. Low levels of testosterone in women are one of the main causes of low libido. Some studies have even shown that testosterone supplements taken by women, especially postmenopausal women, help increase sex drive and sexual sensitivity. It is still in the "testing phase" however, so speak to your OB/GYN about what's available. When being prescribed, make sure to ask about the positive effects and drawbacks and proceed with caution if this is an option you are considering.

The main concern for testosterone supplementation is in women with a family history or other risk factors for heart disease, liver disease, and certain cancers, especially breast cancer. Again, talk with your doctor about what makes sense for you.

If you are a candidate for testosterone supplementation, it is available in synthetic and natural form, from lozenges to creams to suppositories.

quick fix } **MIRROR, MIRROR...**

Remember that episode of *Sex and the City* when her friends challenged Charlotte to get a hand mirror and take a good, long, appreciative look at the part of her that makes her female? Knowing and loving your "lady parts" will help you have better orgasms, and more easily, according to a 2010 study.

GOING *deeper*

Sometimes what affects our sexual interest and enthusiasm is in the here and now, and in those cases, fixing the problem is much less complicated. It's a matter of picking out life's distractions and learning how to block them out. While for some this is a simple process, for others it might take some time to decide what is triggering the distraction.

A Question of Trust

My client, Marianne, a twenty-five-year-old magazine editor, has no trouble having orgasms—it's having them with other people around that's the problem for her. "For as long as I can remember, I can't have an orgasm unless it's me and myself, and, well, my vibrator," she told me. "It's very comfortable and it's very quick. But when I get with a man, I don't know what happens. I just freeze up and I can't let go. It's so frustrating."

"Do you fake orgasms?" I asked her.

"If I really like the guy, yeah, I guess I do," she said. "I don't know what's wrong with me."

In many cases, having "performance anxiety" in the bedroom could stem from a past sexual situation, in which a woman having an orgasm was made to feel uncomfortable about it. It could be something as innocent as her partner laughing at the wrong moment. It could be something more serious and cruel, like a partner who played games with her, bringing her to the brink of orgasm and not always letting her finish. In Marianne's case, the issue probably arose in college. "I lived in a small suite with a few other girls," she said, "and the walls were paper-thin. There was one time I was with my boyfriend back then, and I guess I got a little overzealous. One of my not-so-nice suitemates teased me for weeks," she said. "I had forgotten about that."

I suggested that perhaps her anxiety stems from "getting caught" in the act—which impedes her from "getting too caught up" in it. "When you're by yourself, you have a little more control of the situation," I suggested. "You're in charge of the action, so you know when it's going to wrap, so to speak. You have more of an awareness of what's going on, so you are not as likely to get carried away with things, and you can end whenever you want."

"I guess that makes sense," she said. "But I'd really like to get over this somehow. I really like the guy I'm seeing now, and I'd like to see where we can take our relationship. And I don't want to look back on my life someday and discover that my best lover was my vibrator!"

I explained that by convincing herself she can only have an orgasm by herself, she's making it true, reinforcing that negative association. "You don't talk to that roommate anymore, but you're still letting her get to you," I said. Her trust was shaken, but she was taking it out on the wrong person.

I suggested she bring out her vibrator with her boyfriend and show him how to use it on her by using it on herself. "Invite him to sit back and watch, and while you're pleasuring yourself at first, pretend you're by yourself. As you get more into what you're doing, slowly let yourself know that your partner is there, that he wants you to share this with him, and that he deeply desires to know how he can get it on with you, when you are ready."

Marianne tried my advice with her boyfriend Scott. At first, she wanted him to sit across the room from her, but as she gained his trust, she allowed him on the bed with her, and then to kiss and stroke her while she pleasured herself—and then, ultimately, to take over for her. Once her trust was solidified, she never had another problem having an orgasm with Scott.

Not What I Expected

Julia, a thirty-year-old chef, told me she's given up having orgasms because she's tried every which way and never had one. "All this talk about the earth shaking and the heavens opening and the angels singing—never had that. Not with any of my partners, not with myself."

I wanted to be clear and I asked her: "Are you telling me you never had an orgasm before?"

"I don't know what I've had, but I never had what other people or characters in movies say an orgasm is."

Orgasms are amazing, highly pleasurable sensations, but not all orgasms are equal—and most of the time, the angels do not sing. That doesn't mean you're not having one. And that also doesn't mean you can't be having more powerful ones!

I asked Julia what she felt when she was stimulated sexually. Was there any build, any release?

"I guess I get a little tingling sometimes, but it doesn't last that long."

I explained to her that there are stages of excitement, and that the best way for a woman to have an orgasm is not simply to lie back and let the orgasm happen to her—that an orgasm, for a woman, is something you really go for. Something you actually work for, but not in a bad way.

I explained to her that she could actually increase the intensity and duration of her orgasms with simple movements, breathing techniques, visualizations, and more—which is what the rest of this book is about!

More Serious Concerns

Ellie wrote to me after one of my radio shows and told me she doesn't orgasm and she no longer tries to orgasm. She said all her life, having orgasms has been a hassle and having sex has never been enjoyable, and she wondered if she could just live without the whole package—if she could find a relationship with a man who didn't care about sex and need to have it to be with her.

Without ever meeting Ellie, I could feel something much deeper was going on with her—that her disinterest in sex had more to do with simple boredom or lack of success in having orgasms. That there may have been something that happened to her when she was younger, something perhaps traumatic, that led her to the place where she is now. I wrote to her directly and encouraged her to get help—to call me or see a therapist and get to the root of the issue.

If you are feeling like Ellie, can you pinpoint when your troubles with your libido began? Did it happen overnight, or did you notice a diminishing of drive over time?

If you're struggling to achieve orgasm, if you're getting to the point and not quite getting there during sexual stimulation, is it possible there's an emotional or psychological element at work? Think about it. Can you remember your earliest sexual experiences? Sometimes we carry them with us for the long term, and they can really shape the way we feel about sex.

If you're not comfortable with sex—if you feel guilt, shame, or other negative emotions when it comes to sex—it's possible that your early experiences may have had negative, even painful associations for you that you've been dragging along with you. It may stem from abuse or some other terrible event, and it's not something that's not going to go away by itself. My advice to you is to see a therapist, by yourself or with your partner, and work through it now so you can start enjoying the sex and orgasms you deserve.

Are you suffering from sexual dysfunction? A study conducted by the National Institute of Health in 1999 determined that an overwhelming number of women suffered from some form of sexual dysfunction: 43 percent. Whether those cases were mild or severe was not addressed in the study, but when you consider that almost half of all women are not having sex the way they could and should be, it almost makes you want to scream. And when you consider all the benefits being lost to these women, lost to you, it should really make you want to do something about it! It's essential to get to the heart of the matter and find the solution, whether it's better communication with your partner, or aiding the mechanics of intercourse with lube, devices, or medication. Pills, as we'll discuss in the next section, while being a solution for one person, can bring about even more problems in side effects for another. Even the daily medication we take for seemingly unrelated problems might be having an effect on your sex life.

upper DOWNERS

If you're on antidepressants, such as Prozac or Paxil, they could actually be leveling your sex drive while they're leveling your mood. But it isn't just antidepressants that depress your libido. Birth control pills, blood pressure meds, and almost ironically, certain estrogen-replacement regimens are also known to squash your sexual urges.

That doesn't mean you should go off any of these drugs; you have been prescribed them by your doctor because they are helping you. But you might consider speaking to your doctor about adjusting your dosage or switching from one brand of birth control to the other. Not all things are equal, and how various substances react with your particular body and brain chemistry should be what decides what you take.

Common Drugs That Squash Your Sex Drive

Aldomet. For the lowering of blood pressure and treatment of hypertensio.

Cordarone. For the correction of heart rhythm issues.

Dilantin. For the control of seizures.

Elavil. For the treatment of depression.

Inderal. A beta-blocker that treats angina, tremors, high blood pressure, heart rhythm, and circulation issues.

Lanoxin. For regulating heart rhythm and strengthening heartbeat.

Lithium. For managing the "manic" symptoms of bipolar disorder.

Lopressor. A diuretic that prevents the body from absorbing too much salt.

Nizoral. For treating fungal infections.

Progesterone. For regulation of menstruation and ovulation.

Reglan. For treating heartburn.

Tagamet. For minimizing stomach acid and preventing ulcers.

Tegretol. For controlling seizures.

Valium. For managing anxiety and anxiety disorders.

Zantac. For reduction of stomach acid and prevention and treatment of ulcers.

NO-BRAINER *libido* LIFTERS

There are many small measures you can take to improve sex and your chances of explosive orgasms. Here are just a few quick, easy measures you can take.

Don't smoke.

Not surprising that this would top any list that has to do with healthier living! But the reasons for not smoking when it comes to trying to achieve orgasm are actually pretty specific. Smoking narrows your blood vessels, which means less blood (and all the good stuff in it) getting to the parts that really need it when the mood is right!

Don't over-imbibe.

Having a glass or two of wine to relax yourself and your inhibitions can be a very good thing. But when you take it too far and get yourself plastered, you not only lose awareness of things going on around you, you also lose sensitivity in your body when you want it most!

Eat right.

The old phrase "You are what you eat" really hits home here. As with any area of your life, if you fuel yourself poorly, filling up on processed foods, fatty fast food, sugary substances, and all the things you know are not so good for you, you're going to run out of steam. When you eat right, having a diet of whole foods, adequate protein, natural sugars, and items that really nourish and stay with you, you'll increase your stamina. That's not too hard to see!

Sample all those sensual so-called "sex foods."

Because really, what do you have to lose? No one's saying that foods considered aphrodisiacs are going to create a direct line to sexual satisfaction, but consider some of the foods that are considered aphrodisiacs: the sensuality of raw oysters, the way strawberries can be fed (by you or your lover) with the fingertips, the lusciousness of whipped cream (especially in places it was never intended to belong), the sweetness of chocolate. (Did you know there are chemicals in chocolate that are related to sexual release, tryptophan, which makes up serotonin and phenylethylamine, which is a kind of amphetamine released in the brain when you fall in love?) Also, there are herbs that can get you wet. Black cohosh and dong quoi taken as pill or liquid supplements can actually make you more, well, supple.

Exercise.

We mentioned earlier that just twenty minutes of exercise before sex can pump up the volume on your sexual experience, but consider the stamina you have in all aspects of your life when you exercise regularly. Why should sex be any different?

Feel good about YOU.

Regular exercise makes you feel good because it releases happy endorphins into your blood. It also tones you and helps your clothes fit better, which in turn makes you feel better. Because the best sexual enhancer there is, without question, is self-esteem. When you feel good about yourself, your sex drive and your enjoyment of sex soar; conversely, when you loathe yourself, sex suffers. We're going to get into sex and self-esteem some more as we move through this chapter.

NOW *you* KNOW . . .

Not having orgasms or the kind of orgasms you want to be having does not mean there's anything "wrong" with you, but the situation can escalate, leading to other problems down the road—for your physical and mental health and also your sense of self-esteem and your relationship. Don't let that scare you; rather, let it remind you that having orgasms in your life is as essential to your health and happiness, and even hygiene as, say, brushing your teeth.

Now that you are aware of the main sex-drive squelchers, and are on your way to scaling all walls between you and ecstasy, it's time to get down and dirty! For the rest of the book, we're going to focus on technique—and plenty of it. Because come on, doesn't your life depend on it?

PART TWO

unle

O

p

sh the
ver

Now that you know all the magical goodness orgasms have in store for you, it's time to get some! You should be wanting them daily—and you should be having them that often. If you can find time to take a shower, you can find time to have an orgasm. Hey, you can even have an orgasm in the shower. In this section, we'll show you how, plus give plenty of quick tips for easy ecstasy boosts.

CHAPTER 4

O, THE POSSIBILITIES!

"Freud, as brilliant as he was, defined just two types of female orgasm—vaginal and clitoral. To me, that's like saying the world is flat!"
—ANNIE SPRINKLE, SEX GURU

A former porn star and veritable sexual sage, Annie Sprinkle has been living and breathing sex for a lifetime. So of course, if anyone knows all the other ways to O, and Os that way often, it would be her! But guess what—so can you! And that's what this chapter is all about.

Remember that a woman's most important sex organ exists between our ears and not between our legs. And that even a woman who is paralyzed is able to have an orgasm, thanks to the amazing way her body has been designed by nature. So as orgasms are mostly regulated by our minds, as we now know them to be, can you even imagine how incredibly orgasmic you are as a woman? Think about it. If you can focus your brain to experience and explode with all the sensations, if you can go beyond considering an orgasm as a simple reflex your body has to stimulation and instead embrace it as a beautiful state of mind, just imagine what you can make that mind of yours do for your body? Be prepared, because all the wonderful possibilities in this chapter are sure to astound you!

We all know how powerful our minds can be when it comes to *not* having an orgasm. If we're stressed out about money or the kids, if we're not feeling connected enough to our partner—it's almost impossible to climax when life's problems become obstacles to Os. So . . . who's to say then that can't be turned around? That the power the brain has in controlling our sexual response can't be used for good?

Studies have proven that how a woman feels in and about her relationship directly impacts the power, intensity, and frequency of her orgasms. In studies that used MRI to map a woman's physiological response to orgasm, it was proven that the more in love with her partner a woman was, the stronger and more easily attainable her orgasms. The more she was fully in the moment, engaged in something she truly believed in, the more successful she was at having Os. Makes a lot of sense when you think about it!

In this chapter, we'll get into all the orgasms a woman's body is built to have in illuminating detail. We all know the usual suspects (clitoral, vaginal, G-spot), but what about anal, nipple, or breast? What about orgasms you can have without having any physical contact at all? Read on to embrace all the delicious possibilities!

> Did you know that a warm-up can heat up the intensity of your sexual experience? One study recently proved that engaging in twenty minutes of physical activity prior to sex can amp up your performance and pleasure quotient!

THE BODY *electric*

Annie Sprinkle comments on the studies that have been done about female sexuality: "As important as their research has been, that's like saying LIFE is about heartbeats, blood flow and sweat glands." I couldn't agree with her more. Yes, of course it's important to know the physiology behind how things work. But there is much more to it than just that.

Leah, a listener of one of my radio shows, once called in and asked: "I've heard it's actually possible to have orgasms in places other than 'the usual places.' Is that really true? And if so, do these orgasms feel different than the ones we're used to?"

As I've said, no two orgasms are alike. Each one differs from the next in intensity and duration, though the essence of the sensation is pretty much the same: the amazing tingling and the glorious release. So, when you have orgasms in other places, you still enjoy those wonderful elements of orgasm. How it will feel specifically can vary depending on the place where you experience it.

Always remember an orgasm is controlled by your mind. Know that no matter where you try and experience an orgasm from, it is essential to not just dive in, start stimulating, and then expect to come. Arousal—and for women that means physically, emotionally, and psychologically—is key. The average time for a woman to reach climax is twenty-one minutes. Do you know what the average time for a woman who is fully aroused to reach climax? An amazing three to five minutes! We'll get into more of this as we move through the next chapters of the book, but as you read about all the wonderful ways your body has been hard-wired for pleasure, just know that all the power to have "electric" orgasms rests with you.

When you get good and experienced having orgasms, you're going to find that you will be easier to turn on when the mood strikes—even when the mood isn't quite striking for you but your lover. Take me, for example. I've been having regular orgasms now for a good twenty years—okay, maybe twenty-five years. For me, it doesn't take that long at all to climax, even if I'm not particularly in the mood. Sometimes when my husband wants sex and I may not at that moment (because, like you, I have bills and a kid and other stresses in my life too), I give in. For me, even from that state of "bleh" I can get to "yeah" in a matter of minutes.

I'm not alone in this. I have many friends and clients who are able to turn it on quickly because I and others have trained our brains to be able to turn it on quickly. I've said it before and I'll keep saying it—you have to practice. The more you practice having orgasms (which, happily, means the more you are having orgasms), the more orgasms you will have—and with not a lot of effort or time invested in getting "there." You just have to keep practicing!

THE CLITORAL *o*

The easiest way for most women to orgasm is via stimulation to the clitoris. Of course, this makes perfect sense. Unlike some of the other areas of the female anatomy, the clitoris has one definitive purpose: to make you come. There is nothing else in the history of science that shows that the clitoris is designed to do anything else.

We discussed the clitoris in the first chapter—what it's made up of, how it lies in the vulva, and how it works. Clitoral stimulation can be accomplished in so many ways, and even during intercourse. The methods are broad and really have to do with the individual woman. Some like intense, direct stimulation of the actual clit while others prefer light sweeping motions. And yet, others respond more favorably to stimulation "around the area"—meaning they prefer no direct contact with the clitoris. All of these are normal. All of these are fine. There is no wrong way to stimulate or be stimulated, and we'll get into more of these in the next chapters, which are all about tips and tricks for having orgasms.

Like any orgasm, clitoral orgasms can be mild or intense. The sensation can feel localized to one spot, or they can spread out throughout the body. They can be felt deeply or just on the surface, and they can last anywhere from ten seconds to sixty seconds—and sometimes longer.

Clitoral orgasms can be the only kinds of orgasms a woman has, or they can be a doorway to more kinds. Again, it really depends on the individual woman and what works for her.

My friend, Amanda, a thirty-eight-year-old divorcee, has been with the same partner, Jack, for almost two years. She has confided in me from time to time that he's more adventurous than her in bed and that he's always pushing to try new things. Amanda says that she's open to sexual experiences, but that she's perfectly happy sticking with having clitoral orgasms.

"It seems like Jack is always coming to the bedroom with new ideas," she told me. "Every time he hears about something new, he immediately wants to try it out on me. I'm okay with a lot of the games and the experimenting he likes to try. For instance, the other day he came home with a box of silk scarves and wanted to tie me up. I thought that was cool. I was really turned on by it. Except when he had me all tied up like that, he told me he wanted me to try and make me come another way—with my butt! I wasn't at all comfortable doing that, and he seemed okay with passing on it, at least this time, but also kind of disappointed in me that I didn't want to expand the possibilities. Is there something wrong with me? Do I need to come another way? I'm already very satisfied with how I come. How can I get him to see that?"

I told her, as a professional and a friend, that the only way to get him to see anything was to talk to him about it. "It would be great for you to try new things, of course," I told her. But I also told her that she needs to be as comfortable as possible with sex and what's going on as that's the only way to truly enjoy it. "You only need to come the way you want to," I told her. "So if you are satisfied with the way you're coming now, you have to tell Jack that—and not make him guess it but use actual words. However, don't dismiss what he's trying to accomplish with you when you do. Focus on the positives. Describe to him how you come when he does all the wonderful things he does and how it feels to you. Stress to him that you are really satisfied, and explain just how good things are. And that you may be open to trying new things, but for now, it makes you feel pressured."

Amanda took my advice and had a talk with Jack. He understood and promised to try not to make her feel pressured into attempting more than she was comfortable with doing. And she added something on her own: "I told him that when I felt open to trying different things I would let him know that too. I actually even have some ideas. I feel like now that the pressure's off, I actually have more ideas for some more unconventional things I may want to try."

Then there was another woman, Jessica, who used to call in to my show so frequently we became friends "on the air." Jessica was one of those lucky women who was always able to have effortless orgasms. In fact, climaxing was so easy for her she was stupefied to learn that other women sometimes had trouble getting into the zone. "It's literally like sneezing for me!" she once boasted on a show I was hosting about women who have trouble orgasming (much to the annoyance of the other listeners). I challenged her, playfully: "If you're really such an expert on all of this, why don't you share with the audience all the kinds of orgasms you have—and how you have them?"

"Well," she said, confidently and maybe a little smugly, "I try, no matter what position I'm in, to always make sure I'm getting lots and lots of clitoral stimulation. In fact, if I really want to come quickly, I get on top, lean way forward, and rub up against my boyfriend while he's inside me. I also rock my pelvis quite vigorously."

"That's good advice," I said. "But how do you have other kinds of orgasms? All the other kinds?"

"All the other kinds?" she asked. "Oh, I get it. You mean like intense or prolonged or just slightly tingly or—"

"No," I challenged. "I mean, *where* do you have your other orgasms. Are they vaginal? Anal? Do you have cervical orgasms?"

She paused briefly and then replied, "Just from my clitoris, I guess."

I decided to have a little fun with my friend. "You mean you never had an orgasm by being stimulated in any other place aside from your clit?"

"Uh . . . no. I guess I haven't."

"Great!" I said. "Then the next show I do will be for you. Because you're actually missing out on a whole world of orgasming and I think it's going to blow your mind!"

And now I'm going to blow yours.

THE VAGINAL *o*

There is a school of thought that believes that a vaginal orgasm is simply a clitoral orgasm, expanded. Remember that the clitoris extends (think of that "wishbone" image) down from the "top." Some believe that a vaginal orgasm then is just sensation stemming down from the main area.

But remember all those nerves we talked about that are actually in the vagina, at least in the lower third, working from the entrance in? For some women, this patch of nerves is about so much more than feeling the penis of their partners entering and exiting them. For some women, when this area is stimulated during penetration, orgasm is possible. Remember that a small number of women are able to orgasm through sex alone without any further stimulation? This is why.

In my work, I have uncovered all kinds of interesting Os that women have been able to have, and I firmly believe you can learn to have any type of orgasm you want. For some, an orgasm is as simple as an automatic response; for others, it's more of a learned response.

To *learn* how to have a vaginal O, an orgasm generated from the vaginal area and cervix, I recommend plenty of self-stimulation. We'll get deeper into this in the next chapter, but I'll give you a taste here.

When you pleasure yourself, avoid any contact whatsoever with your clitoris. I want you to get to know your vagina here. When you touch yourself, focus on the vaginal canal and try to find your G-spot (see page 80).

Also, pay attention to your AFE zone (the anterior fornix erogenous zone), the deepest part of the vagina, which is located past the G-Spot and above the cervix, where the vagina begins to curve. You can find it by inserting a finger or two along the upper wall, reaching the deepest point. Consider that the vaginal canal is only about three inches long, which is not as long as most of your fingers. Insert your finger or fingers into your vagina, and push up gently until you find your cervix. You'll know you got to it as it will feel rounder and firmer than the rest of your vagina. Just above the cervix is the A.F.E. Zone, which will feel somewhat spongy.

Press the A.F.E. Zone. Massage it and see if it feels good for you. Do you feel any extra lubrication coming from this area? The A.F.E. is in charge of lubricating your vagina.

Massage your G-spot and this area one after another and see if you can't have a vaginal orgasm from one or both of these areas.

quickfix } **SPECIAL TIPS FOR VAGINAL O'S**

- Self-pleasure with your fingers first and stimulate the first third of the vagina. Insert your well-lubed fingers inside and out and round and round.

- Next, using a vibrating bullet, continue the same stimulation. Go back and forth from your fingers and then the bullet and no matter how tempted you are to stimulate your clitoris, don't do it! Practice this regularly for a minimum of a month or until you learn how to become vaginally sensitive.
- Now, stimulate your G-spot with your fingers or a toy. Again, avoid contact with your clitoris, something you'll want to do until you've learned to turn these other areas into orgasmic hot spots. It takes practice, but it can be done!
- During intercourse, have your partner aim his penis so that he ends up massaging your G-spot.
- Doing Kegels during sex can increase vaginal Os.
- Lying on your back, insert a six-inch smooth vibe, like a My First Vibe, into your vagina and turn it on. Then just relax. Don't move at all, and see how this can awaken your vagina as you lie back and feel the sensations and think about what you are feeling and *how* it's feeling.
- Try incorporating more foreplay on the interior of your vagina before intercourse. The stimulation may increase your chances of having a vaginal O.

THE G-SPOT *O*

The G-spot orgasm is a source of almost constant controversy. Some sex researchers believe it doesn't exist. Some believe it's one of the most significant types of orgasm a woman can have. Then there's the buzz surrounding the G-Spot orgasm right in the bedroom. Some women have never had one and feel distressed that they haven't. Others have almost had them, but panicked because they felt just as the orgasm was beginning to crest that they were going to pee all over their partner! And then there's the actual secretion issue that freaks women out. Yes, there are women who can ejaculate. And yes, it is not as common as other reactions to orgasm. But it is perfectly natural and can be wonderful. It's not weird; it's "special." But we'll get into that more in a bit. First, let's get into the G-spot itself.

The G-Spot, short for the Grafenberg spot, was first discovered in the 1940s by German gynecologist Dr. Ernst Grafenberg, who was conducting studies having to do with the difference between urethra stimulation and stimulation of the vaginal wall. What Dr. Grafenberg learned was that there was indeed something going on right there inside the vagina, but on the opposite wall. While it could be felt through the vagina, this area, this bean-shaped spot, was actually something separate and that when stimulated it could spark orgasms in women. Dr. Grafenberg felt that he had stumbled onto something big, but it wasn't until the 1980s that his discovery got a name.

Since then, there's been almost constant speculation surrounding this area, with some scientists and researchers believing it to be part of the vagina while others guess it's a component of the clitoris. Some have worried that the existence of the G-Spot could put another level of pressure and stress on women to have orgasms (like Amanda), complicating their lives instead of enhancing them. Still others have taken the stance that there is no such thing as a G-Spot, and to insist that there is one only allows sexual impresarios to take advantage of the masses by promising a new technique that could never work. These people have never had a G-Spot orgasm.

Like anything else I'll teach you in this book, this orgasmic experience is something that can be absolutely awesome if you are open to it. If you're not, that's okay. It's not a matter of "You haven't lived until you've had a G-Spot orgasm!" Not by a long shot. But if you want to try it, know that the G-Spot does exist (it's been coined the "female prostate"; ironically the prostate in males has been coined "the male G-Spot"), it's incredibly sensitive, and you may have to push against your normal levels of comfort to achieve it.

In order to achieve a G-Spot orgasm, direct, firm penetration is essential. Remember that you access the G-Spot via the vagina around two or so inches inside toward the upper front wall—but it's buried in that wall about a centimeter. So while a light grazing over your clitoris may be stimulation enough, it isn't going to work to get a G-Spot orgasm. Whether you or your partner uses a finger (or two) or a special G-Spot vibrator, a device with a specially curved tip designed to hit up right against the right spot when inserted, firm pressure is key! We'll get into more specific techniques as we move through this book.

Wet and Wild.

Alexa called in to my radio show and told me: "I waited a long time to have sex with my new boyfriend and then when we finally did I forgot to tell him that sometimes I squirt. I'm one of those women who female ejaculates. When it happened he was so stunned and I think he thinks I peed on him. How can I explain this to him? We haven't said much about it and we haven't had sex again either."

Here's the thing about a G-Spot orgasm: Sometimes it causes a phenomenon known as "gushing" or "squirting." What it really is, is something known as female ejaculation. It happens to a fair number of women, it has to do with G-Spot stimulation, and it absolutely, positively is not peeing. Though women sometimes worry that it is because the pressure that builds just before a G-Spot orgasm is quite similar to the pressure you feel just before you have to pee, and the release it causes may feel as if you have.

I told Alexa that first and foremost, it was important that this not be a "surprise" for her boyfriend—that she explain to him what was going on beforehand. I also told her that if he had any questions, they could look it up together. I can save some of you that trouble here!

Female ejaculate is not urine. Like the guys' version, the stuff that comes out of us has traces of urine, but this is simply due to the path it travels (think about it). It's actually more like semen than anything else, though also distinct in and of itself. Essentially, it's fluid produced by the paraurethra glands, also known as the "Skenes glands." In small quantities, it's mucouslike, but the more that comes out, the clearer and thinner it becomes.

During G-spot stimulation, the surrounding tissue expands thanks to the fluid, and the orgasmic release simply releases that fluid.

The volume of liquid released has also been known to shock a lover or two. Janelle wrote to me about it for one of my columns: "Do you have any tips for controlling how wet my mattress gets?!"

I do! There are actually products available for just this kind of thing. (See resources.) I won't get into them specifically here, but there are waterproof, easily cleaned throw blankets, mats, and even covered pillows (that can also be positioned to enhance the experience) that can help you keep this somewhat slippery situation under control. You could also purchase a waterproof mattress pad to make your life easy!

Whatever you decide, don't let a little liquid come between you and experiencing one of the most amazing Os possible!

THE CERVICAL *o*

The cervix is the gateway to the uterus—and also a potential gateway to pleasure if manipulated correctly! And as the deepest part of the vagina, it's also where you can experience your deepest orgasms. But most women have never considered this to be an orgasmic place. Why?

For one, especially for women who have had babies, we come to think of it as a gauge of sorts—"Her cervix is dilated four centimeters!" Sometimes it has to do with improper cervix stimulation. Certainly we've all been there when our partner achieves incredibly deep penetration, bangs the head of his penis against our cervix, and all we can think is *ouch!* But there's a reason you feel that banging so intensely: The cervix is embedded with lots of luscious nerve endings and, when properly stimulated, can produce an orgasm like no other.

We may think we just invented this idea that the cervix can be an orgasm zone, but it's something the ancients knew and took full advantage of. Don't believe me? Take a look at some of the descriptions and illustrations in the *Kama Sutra* and tell me there wasn't any motive for some of those crazy positions that allowed for some crazy-deep penetration!

Anne was a client of mine who was interested in experimenting with cervical orgasms because she was sure she had had one before. "It was not like any other orgasm I ever had," she explained. "It was really intense and deep, and happened more in my lower abdomen. Higher than usual. It felt awesome," she said, "but I have no idea how I managed to have it—and how I can have another one like it."

I asked if she was sure it was cervical—that it wasn't an orgasm from her G-spot or clitoris. "No way," she assured. "I've definitely had those kinds of orgasms before and this was definitely unlike anything I had ever experienced before."

So Anne and I talked the experience through, trying to find out just what it was that triggered such a different sensation in her. "I remember it was after my boyfriend and I had been going at it for a while. I remember being really revved up and wet, and whatever he was doing, well, he did it just right. Except we're not together anymore," she said.

"Not to worry," I assured her. "You can try to find it yourself again with a 'Realistic'—a dildo that resembles your ex's member." (And yes, they do make dildos that look incredibly real, and they are actually called "Realistics.") Because they're perceived as being "graphic," they're generally kept behind the counter in stores—you have to ask to see them.

"When you get your Realistic, resist the urge to use it right away," I told her. "Be sure to pleasure yourself first, with your fingers or even a vibrator, and get yourself nice and wet and ready. Then take the Realistic and insert it. Use the Realistic to lightly tap around your cervix to try and discover what feels good and what doesn't."

Anne got her Realistic and then got to work. A couple of weeks later, she reported back to me that she had found success. "At first it didn't work out so well," she said. "I jabbed myself a couple of times and it didn't feel that good when I hit the top or middle of my cervix. But then I repositioned my new 'friend' so that it hit the bottom of my cervix, and it felt good—amazing even."

A few months later, Anne got a new boyfriend, and as soon as she was comfortable doing so, she showed him, with the Realistic, just what to do with his own member. It worked like a charm. "During sex, he sometimes aims for this area, which is kind of hard to hit sometimes, but he tries—and when he does hit it, it feels just wonderful!"

The best positions in intercourse for a woman to have a cervical O are the ones in which the deepest penetration is possible. Woman on top works wonders. Missionary could also work, with a pillow resting underneath her behind to shift her angle properly. We'll look at more possibilities in later chapters when we get into positions and variations, but the most important thing to remember is a question of "thrust." It's essential that the thrusting is neither too fast or aggressive. The penis should tap lightly against the cervix, not crash into it!

quick fix } **TIPS FOR HAVING CERVICAL Os**

- Have your partner gently aim for the bottom of your cervix during sex.
- Using a vibrator or dildo, lightly tap various areas of your cervix to see if it feels enjoyable.
- Be sure to find your own comfort zone. Most women I know find it more comfortable for the lower part of the cervix to be stimulated than the top or middle.

ANAL *o*

Like the vagina, the anus is also loaded with nerve endings, and for women and men, these nerve endings can create an environment for orgasms to flourish. Most experts believe, however, that anal Os are brought about because of the anus's proximity to the clitoris in females and the prostate in males.

Remember that the clitoris extends (there's that wishbone again) down, and the edges of it lie close to the anus, which means increased sensitivity for females.

If you're not comfortable with anal play, that's okay. It's not for everyone. Also, only a small percentage of women are able to have an orgasm from anal sex alone. It's not easy, but it's not impossible. Though it's more common that a woman will have an anal orgasm through anal play. Also, in many cases, anal play is a catalyst for other kinds of orgasms.

Cheryl was a woman who used to call in to my show often. She admitted she liked to have anal sex sometimes, and when she did, she always had a great orgasm from it. One day, I asked her to share what she knew with the rest of the audience and to give them some tips on how to have great anal orgasms.

"I don't exactly love anal," she said, "but my boyfriend likes it, so I do sometimes give in. He's very gentle, and we always use a condom and plenty of lube. Basically, we do it 'doggie-style,' but with me in complete control of the situation."

She continued to tell the audience that she remained in control the entire time and communicated verbally any time he needed to know something: slower, faster, ouch that hurts, stop, go, etc. "But my orgasm didn't really come on from any of this," she said. "What really brought it on was thinking of how nasty I was being—how I was such a bad, bad girl for letting my man do this to me. The more I thought about it, the more excited I got. So really, it wasn't a matter of positioning or in and out, or any physical stimulation of any kind." What got Cheryl off during anal sex was a stimulation of the mind.

"It only took minutes of thinking to get me off," she said. "I start orgasming like crazy and it feels clitoral—but I can feel it everywhere!"

Know the Risks

Anal sex can be wonderful when it's handled correctly, but it is considered a pretty risky behavior by the CDC (Center for Disease Control). Whatever you do, don't engage in it lightly. Read about it with your partner first, know the risks and talk them through. Here are some things you should know, from a CDC fact sheet:

- Condoms are more likely to break during anal sex than during vaginal intercourse. For that reason, you need to be extra cautious. Be sure the lube you are using will not degrade the condom (see page 52) and be sure to use enough that you create a very slippery entry.

· The thin lining of the rectum is more prone to allowing the HIV virus to enter the body, so it is so important to know your lover and your lover's sexual history well. You may even decide to each get tested for HIV before embarking on anal sex.

· Never have anal sex while intoxicated or under the influence of drugs. If you can't be in control of yourself, you can't be in control of the situation.

· Take it slow. Start by inserting a finger first, and then a smaller toy. Work your way up in size.

· Always use plenty of lube. Slipping and sliding is what it's all about here. The less lube there is, the more chance there is of tearing a condom and even the delicate tissues of the anus, causing anal fissures.

BREAST AND NIPPLE *O*'S

Have you ever had a friend tell you that she could have an orgasm just by having her breasts and nipples played with? Or is this something that has happened to you?

My client, Sheila, came to me one day after sharing cocktails and girl talk with a coworker and couldn't believe what the other woman had told her. "Beth has a tendency to exaggerate, if you know what I mean," said Sheila. "She always inflates her contributions around the office and seems to take more credit for what her team gets accomplished than what I think is warranted. So when she told me after a few Cosmos that she only needed to have her boobs played with to come, I of course believed she was full of it. But when I asked some other friends, some said that they had had the same experience, while others were in my camp: That this was a total lie. Is it possible to have an orgasm if only your nipples and breasts are stimulated?"

Of course! It may not happen all the time, but when you consider all the ingredients needed for an orgasm—nerve endings, stimulation, and a mindset ready to "take it"—it makes complete sense that this would be possible.

Some people have very sensitive nipples, and many attest to the fact that having their nipples stimulated—kissed, stroked, squeezed—can enhance their orgasms when other factors are at work; namely, that they or their partner is paying amorous attention to their nether regions with a hand or sex toy (or, in the case of there being a partner present, mouth, lips, and tongue). Having a nipple orgasm, sometimes playfully referred to as a "nipplegasm," requires concentration and focus—of using that sexy brain of yours to place all the orgasmic emphasis on your nipples and breasts as you can. If your brain is focusing on those things that get you off while your nipples are being played with, you may actually be able to forge a subconscious connection between the two and eventually you will begin to climax simply through the stimulation of your nipples and breasts!

So, in reality, this may be more of a "sensory O" (see below), but it is an orgasm you can attain all the same. I'll give you some tips and tricks as we move through the other chapters in this book. (Oh, and just as a side note, some men have very sensitive nipples too, so one thing you might try with your partner is treating each other to nipplegasms the next time you're looking to try something new and adventurous between the sheets.)

SENSORY *O*

Some women can be touched everywhere but the obvious orgasm hot spots and reach orgasm—just like we covered above in breast and nipple Os. Instead of an orgasm concentrated on a small area, they use their brains and their orgasmic focus to have an orgasm just by being touched.

This has actually happened to me during a massage. There I was on the table having all the stress and strains of my life kneaded out of me by a pair of very skilled, firm hands. While the tension was being released, I could feel another release rising within me—an orgasmic release. I actually had an orgasm, lying on my tummy, right there on the massage table. It was amazing! Of course I didn't tell the person who had been working on me what happened. I tried to cover it up by pretending to sneeze and then squiggled around after it happened. It may have been a little embarrassing, but I was thrilled to know, for myself, that it was possible. I even asked around—friends and clients—and learned that similar things had happened to others, that other women have been able to experience orgasm without having any of the usual places stimulated. It's rare, but it's not impossible, and we'll get deeper into this as we go along.

"Microgasms"

Annie Sprinkle is a proponent of the of the sensory O, and believes they can happen daily on a smaller scale. She calls these types of Sensory O's "Microgasms" and, according to Annie, "Orgasm is within us . . . If we simply stop and focus on our erotic body energy , and visualize the orgasmic flow inside of us, we can physically feel orgasmic waves pulse through our bodies and feel the 'tension and release' on a very subtle level." She goes on to explain that we can channel a sneeze into an orgasm. Even if we get the chills, we can refocus that. If we experience something pleasurable, we can rewire ourselves to experience these things orgasmically—the sun on our face, the wind in our hair. She says of these "microorgasms": "They reside just below our surface. All we need to do is let them bubble up."

multiples!

Are multiple orgasms real or not? Some people say they don't exist, but maybe this is because they don't quite understand what multiple orgasms are. For example, my client Liz told me, "Sometimes I'll have an orgasm during foreplay, which is usually by oral or fingering, then I have intercourse with my partner and I have another orgasm. Is this a multiple orgasm or do they have to be one after the other?"

I explained to Liz that in fact, yes, she was having multiple orgasms. Sometimes people think that having multiple orgasms mean they come one right after the other, in rapid succession. That after your release, another builds and happens directly after it. That has been known to happen, but it's more common that you will be able to have more than one orgasm over the course of a sexual session, like Liz, meaning one from foreplay, maybe one during sex, maybe one after sex.

But multiples can be a lot more fun than even that! We've learned all the many ways our bodies can experience orgasms—and we've learned that we can have them one right after the other. But what if multiple orgasms happened with different types of orgasms? Annie Sprinkle explains: "Sometimes a gal has just one kind of orgasm in one part of the body, in one way. But often two or more kinds of orgasm are combined in succession or in tandem. These can be in absolutely any combination. During a single sex session, one might experience them all." Talk about bliss!

NOW *you* KNOW

While as a woman you have a special organ specially designed for providing you with sexual pleasure, it is far from the only hot button for happiness that exists within you! Thanks to your amazing brain and a network of nerve endings just waiting to be repurposed for your pleasure, you can have orgasms in places and ways you may never before dreamed possible—by yourself or with a partner. The rest of this book will give you the tips and techniques you need to maximize your pleasure!

CHAPTER 5

GETTING TO *know* YOU

"*Women do not take longer to orgasm than men . . . The majority of the women in Kinsey's study masturbated to orgasm within four minutes, similar to the men in this study.*"

—SHERE HITE, FAMED SEX RESEARCHER

G ot a headache? Go have an orgasm! Feeling anxious or depressed or blue? Treat yourself to a sweet release and let that oxytocin surge right through you!

Now that we've covered most of the health benefits—physical, mental, and emotional—of orgasms for women, and we've explored all kinds of orgasm options there are to have, it's time to get to the good part. The actual *getting yours* part.

Remember that it's all about frequency. The more orgasms you have, the more you *will* have, and the more you practice having orgasms, the easier they will come to you. So you need to make having an orgasm part of your daily routine, like brushing your teeth. And you need to get your daily dose of Vitamin O whether you are with someone else or alone.

Relying on yourself is a great way to ensure you get your daily dose of O because even if your partner is working late, away on business, or just out playing golf, you can still get what you need. Your private time will enhance your couple time. As you become more intimate and aware of those parts of your body that trigger sweet sensations, you'll learn more about what you like and what you don't. This self-awareness will allow you to better express your needs to your partner. Pleasuring yourself won't take away from the orgasms you can have later with your partner. It will only make them better because before you can have mind-blowing orgasms with a partner, you have to learn how to have them yourself.

You can't show anyone else how to give you what you want if you don't know yourself. In this hugely important chapter, we'll explore all your beautiful explosive parts and get into self-pleasuring techniques. We'll uncover pleasure techniques for one of your most important sex organs—your brain—and even open ourselves to the possibility of having an orgasm without ever laying a hand on ourselves. We'll also talk about "tools", devices you can use to bring on the bliss, which encompass everything from vibrators to dildos to otherwise innocent household items like pillows and vegetables. We'll learn to clear our minds of clutter, free our souls of inhibitions, and unleash the power of our bodies to get the *nourishment* we need—and leave us gasping for more.

> ## quick fix } **MASSAGE THERAPY**
>
> Why not treat yourself to your own "happy ending" the next time you come home from a massage? Thanks to all the touching and rubbing you'll have gotten from the masseuse, you'll probably already be more than halfway there!

GETTING TO KNOW *me*

We've already looked at many of the reasons women don't have orgasms—or have enough of them, but I wanted to save the frustration that women sometimes feel over not being able to orgasm as quickly or easily as they'd like to here.

I was introduced to Meaghan through a mutual friend. The mother of two Meg, lived in a beautiful house in a posh suburb and, on the surface, appeared to have everything she ever wanted. But something was missing in her life, and that's why she came to see me.

"I never have orgasms," she told me.

"Do you mean you never have orgasms with your partner?"

"Yes," she said, sadly.

"What about with yourself?" I asked her. "Do you have orgasms when you masturbate?"

"Masturbate? I don't do that."

"Why?" I asked.

She took a deep breath. "I don't like playing with myself," she explained, "because I can't have an orgasm even then so I don't see the point."

I assured her that many women at one point or another in their lives can have difficulty climaxing, but I also encouraged her to keep trying. "It may seem pointless at first, but you have to try new things. I promise you will find the technique that works for you. And when you do, you can share what you've learned about yourself with your partner. But you should take some time to get to know yourself first—so you know what to share."

I assured Meg that just like with anything else, the more she "practiced" the better she'd get at it, and eventually, she would know just what techniques and patterns worked for her. A few weeks later, after much "practicing," Meg called, happy to report that she may have discovered what works for her.

Of course, self-pleasuring is not the only way to have an orgasm, but it's a great place to start. It would be ridiculous to wake up one morning and believe you have the ability to ride a bike if you never rode a bike before. The same is true with orgasming. You aren't going to magically wake up one day and just have it down if you never did it before. You have to teach your body how to respond organically. You have to teach yourself how to *become* orgasmic.

The reason that self-pleasuring is a great place to start is that it takes the pressure off. When it's just you, you can really take your time getting to where you need to be. You can take away the element of "stage fright," relax, and leisurely figure it all out for yourself. Some days you might get close and not quite clinch it. Other days you might just get there. You may also just enjoy the sensations of self-exploration—of doting on yourself.

Just keep trying everything. Experiment with different types of stimulation, experiment with toys, and by all means practice everything you read in this book! Because like Meg, all you really need is a little confidence, a little faith, and a little knowledge about how your body works, and you'll be well on your way!

orgasm 101

One of the reasons women don't have orgasms is that they don't really understand how to have orgasms. There are basically two phases of orgasm: rev and release. The first is the build, the next is the rush; but you need to be aware of yourself, your body, and how you are responding to all the things happening to you.

First, the Rev. There's a line of thinking some women have that they are simply just supposed to lie back and let an orgasm happen to them. If this is how you think, you have to disabuse yourself of that—and quickly. Having an orgasm is not a passive event. It's an active endeavor that calls on your mind and your body. If your car won't start, do you just sit there and will it to ? Or do you rev the engine and actively make it start? The same holds true here.

For your mind, the keyword is focus. Try and put your brain in a place where you can actually have this orgasm. Thinking about a permission slip you need to sign is not the right place. Mentally mapping out your grocery list is not the right place. Think of sexy things. Fantasize. Visualize. There should be no one else in the world but you.

For your body, please, please, please don't just lie there. Find a rhythm that works for you. Tilt your hips. Gyrate. Move into the source of pleasure. Use your free hand to stroke the rest of you.

Don't just relax while you're lying there pleasuring yourself. Tense up. Muscle tension and release is what orgasm is all about, so don't be afraid to tense up. Do your Kegels! When you tense up those muscles down in your legs and buttocks and tummy, you're also increasing the blood flow to these regions. Increased blood flow means greater sensitivity, and greater sensitivity means—you guessed it—greater orgasms!

Once you get yourself all worked up, it's time for the second part. The amazing part. The release.

Again, just don't lie there. When you feel an orgasm coming, help it along. Adjust your breathing. Deeper, fuller breaths. Breathe in and out through your mouth and nose. And if the mood strikes, let yourself cry out when an orgasm takes you over. Don't hold back.

Remember: The more of yourself you put into an orgasm, the more you're going to get out of it!

WILL YOU STILL LOVE *me* IN THE MORNING?

When we make love to our partners, we treat them with kisses and sweet caresses. We make them feel like there is no one more special in the world than they are. So why wouldn't we also want the same for ourselves when we make love to ourselves? Sure, it's not possible to actually make out with yourself, but that doesn't mean we can't still remind ourselves of how special we are.

Write "I love me" on a sheet of paper and tape it over your bed. Repeat the phrase over and over again while you're self-pleasuring, in your mind, even out loud and proud. Remind yourself that there's no one in the world who deserves the exquisite pleasure you're about to bestow on yourself more than you.

MIND *over* THE MUNDANE

A man could orgasm in a burning house; we're wired differently. Even the slightest distraction can throw us off course. While our brains can be a wonderful asset to us when it comes to coming—think fantasy!—they can also ruin the party if there's too much going on up there. So before you do anything else, take the time to get yourself in the right frame of mind.

- *If you can't relax, you can't release.* Turn off the phone and the computer and the BlackBerry—or at least turn them down so you can't hear them. Not having to worry about interruptions will get you there quicker. Lock the door, pull down the shades, whatever it takes for you to give you the privacy and seclusion you need to just let go.

- *Attitude is everything.* Whether you're by yourself or with your partner, from this point on you are not allowed to say "I just can't have an orgasm" or "This isn't going to work." Banish all those negative thoughts and keep repeating this mantra in your head: "I come easily and frequently, I come easily and frequently, I come easily and frequently . . ."

- *Take away the pressure.* Orgasms get better and better the more we have them, so if the earth doesn't shake when you're just starting out, so what. You wouldn't expect to run a marathon the first time you take a jog. Little tremors are just as enjoyable—and just as effective for all the benefits O provides.

- *Set the mood.* If you want to light some candles or incense, go ahead. If you want to build a fire in the fireplace, or lay out on some soft pillows on the floor, knock yourself out. Play music on your DVD player or iPod, or even sounds from the beach. Adjust your surroundings in whatever way you see fit to help you get your mind in the right place.

- *Dress—or undress—the part.* Sometimes wearing something sexy and lacy and silky will enhance your experience, and sometimes wearing nothing at all is the way to go. I have a friend who likes to pleasure herself with a pocket rocket right over her tightest jeans—without undoing the zipper or anything. It's all about what gets *you* going.

- *Batteries not required.* Though they might be requested. A vibrator or other tool is a great thing to have on hand, especially if time is limited. And depending on what technique you choose to use, be sure to have a bottle of lube close by.

OUT OF MIND, *into* BODY

What woman on the planet doesn't ruminate over things constantly, even when it's time for sex? Even I'm guilty of it! But the more time we spend in the wrong places in our minds, the harder it becomes to get aroused and to climax.

Your goal then, before trying to have an orgasm, is mindfulness. A state of awareness in practice by Eastern philosophies for centuries, mindfulness means simply existing in full awareness and in the present moment. When you're in that moment, you are acutely aware of everything that exists only in that moment (your breathing, your heartbeat) and nothing that does not exist in the moment—your job, your mortgage, and that kind of thing.

Even though your mind is what's going to get you over the finish line, you almost have to pull out of it to stay in the race! And block out the parts of it that don't matter in the moment. You have to put your complete focus on, well, the task at hand.

Meditation is a popular way to achieve mindfulness. Try this meditation exercise the next time you're wondering if you paid the water bill or signed your kid's report card while you're getting "busy" with your partner or yourself.

1. *First, find a comfortable spot.*

Whether you're sitting in a chair or on the floor, or lying down on your bed, you want to make sure that nothing is going to distract you: like the hard arm of a dining room chair jabbing you in the rib, or not having enough support sitting on a backless stool (or worrying about falling off if you get too relaxed!).

2. *Next, make yourself comfortable.*

Wear loose clothing—or no clothing at all if that's what works for you. Being constantly reminded that you need to take off a couple of pounds because the button on the waistline of your jeans keeps stabbing you or you're wearing underwear that tends to "climb" into your nether regions is going to take away from your ability to focus.

3. *Then, close your eyes.*

Physically block out the world by blocking your visual access to it. (You might also consider putting some quiet music on your iPod and blocking out your audible access to the world as well. Nothing kills concentration like the sound of a truck backing up or the neighborhood kids fighting outside.)

4. *Now, take charge of your brain.*

Imagine yourself like a cowboy, or something along those lines, taking all the wild ideas racing through your head and rounding them up with your lasso, then corralling them somewhere else for a while. You know they aren't going away—but at least you can set them aside for now, and keep them contained so they don't come crashing in on your moment.

5. *And focus.*

I want you to focus on one simple idea: pleasure. Think about the word and what it means to you.

See it spelled out in your head, letter by letter.

Sound it out in your brain—say it to yourself over and over. Take it slow and really listen to every sound there is to be heard in this word.

Silently mouth it, and feel each sound in your mouth. How is your mouth moving around the sounds? It's actually a very sexy word to say when you focus so intently on it like this.

Imagine what the word tastes like, and what it smells like.

Imagine the word wrapping itself around your body, like your favorite blanket or robe. Warming you. Soothing you. Enveloping you.

6. *And maintain.*

You want to try and focus like this for about thirty minutes, but you may have to work up to that. The last thing you want to be doing is stressing yourself out because you have an egg timer ticking away next to you and you're pulling out of your zone worrying that you aren't spending enough time in it! Start without timing yourself at all. Maybe you go a minute—and then five. Eventually, the more you practice, you'll get to thirty minutes, and even beyond that. Just like anything else, the more you do it, the more natural it will feel to you, and the better you will become at it.

EXPLORING *your* OPTIONS

Let's review: the clitoris contains more than six thousand nerve endings. The nerve endings stretch out from the tip of the clitoris and extend across your lower regions, so why not extend them further in your mind, right to the very tips of your fingers and toes?

As a woman, you are wholly orgasmic. Your brain is a sex organ, and so is your skin. While the center of your sexuality lies between your legs, it stretches out everywhere else. So before you pull out that vibrator or start stimulating yourself down there, I want you to take some time to awaken the rest of you.

Lie on your back and relax. Now, with the tips of your fingers, lightly stroke the top of your other hand, from your wrist to your fingertips. Turn over your hand and lightly caress your palm and the inside of your wrist. (Starting to feel the tingles yet? Good!)

Taking longer strokes, run those fingers up the inside of your arm, right up to the elbow, then past the elbow, and all the way up to your shoulder. Run your fingers across your neck and collarbone, stroking between one shoulder and the other. Lightly graze your breasts, and your nipples, and then stop.

Take those fingers and head down with them—all the way down. Now take both hands and lightly run those fingers against your outer legs. Circle around to your inner legs. Stroke up and down between your knees and your pelvis—but do not touch anything in your pelvic region yet. Lightly stroke up and down and enjoy the feeling of your skin coming to life. Then stop.

Now take those fingertips and run them up and down the sides of your torso and all over your tummy. By this point, your sexual "center" should be anxiously awaiting its turn with those magic fingertips of yours. Feel free to give it what it wants, or continue stroking and teasing yourself first, running your fingers over your breast and tummy, around your pelvic region—really giving yourself a good long tease. Next, we'll talk about techniques for stimulation down there.

pleasure PRINCIPLES

As you get to know you a little better, you'll see there is no wrong way to pleasure yourself—only a lot of right ways. Here I'll give you some methods some women use to get to their own pleasure zones. You can follow the directions here to a T, you can use them as a guide and vary them to suit your needs, or you can simply lie back, lube yourself up, and simply explore and enjoy!

Indirect Stimulation

If you find direct stimulation of your clit to be too intense or even painful, don't do it. You don't need to touch your clit directly to have an orgasm. Stimulate around the area instead. After applying some lube (from your own saliva or from a tube), use your index finger and middle finger from both hands together and rub all around your labia, without ever touching your clit. Test both sides to see if you are more sensitive on the right or left side. Experiment with temperature: Rub your hands together first to bring on the heat; introduce an ice cube to chill out. Rubbing outside your panties—even outside your clothes—is also a great way to stimulate without touching.

Direct Stimulation

Some women can go right into direct stimulation of the clitoris, and some need to be warmed up to it. If you're the "dive right in" kind of gal, by all means get right to the point. Use your fingers or just the tips, or use the palm of your hand as you rub, massage, or even lightly flick or tap. As you get closer to orgasm you might find a hot spot to focus on that will bring on your orgasm quicker. Be sure you're paying attention to where it is so you can go right for this spot the next time you're pressed for time and need release at the touch of a button.

Stimulation with Penetration

Some women like the fantasy of having someone else in the room with them, and some women simply like the intensity of feeling penetration when having an orgasm. Penetration during masturbation can also bring on powerful G-Spot orgasms.

As you stimulate your clit and surrounding area with one hand, penetrate your vagina or anus—or both, if you're feeling particularly ambitious—with the other. Just don't forget to use plenty of lube, especially when it comes to your butt. (You could also use a toy, like a vibrator, dildo, or butt plug, but we'll get into that in just a bit.)

Sometimes it's easier to reach everything when you lie on your back with your legs apart. Sometimes you can intensify the sensation when you lie on your tummy and add the weight of your body into the pressure you apply. Whether you're standing, kneeling, sitting in a chair with your legs each comfortably resting over an arm of a chair—it's all about what feels good for you.

> There are many sex toys out there designed with a special "hook" for G-spot stimulation, including the Amore G-spot vibrator. (See resources.)

Bump and Grind

You don't need your fingers or hands to masturbate—especially if what really gets you going is the simulation of actually being in the act. "Rock and roll" with a pillow or blanket between your legs. Straddle the edge of your bed or another piece of furniture. Basically, this is like simulating the "woman on top" sex position, so whatever you like to do in that position, and whatever motion and speed works for you to get the stimulation you need, go for it!

With a Vibrator or Other Device

If Vitamin O is the supplement you need to get your life force flowing, the vibrator is the number one facilitator to your engines going! In the previous chapter, I introduced you to many of the types of vibrators out there. Here, I'm going to start showing you how to use them. One of my favorite vibes for self-pleasuring is the Pocket Rocket, because it's small and discreet, and oh so powerful.

Turn on your Pocket Rocket and run just the tip up and down your labia—inner and outer. Continue pressing the vibe up against the right side of your clit and then the left. Repeat as necessary, varying the order of areas you stimulate. It won't be long till you explode in orgasmic bliss!

If you find the sound of a vibrator distracting, turn on some music or place a pillow over the device and the area you're using it on. You can also opt for a silent toy, like a dildo. Here's a fun way to use a dildo, especially if you're a fan of "bump and grind": Prop up the dildo between two stacks of pillows and ride it on home. Let your fantasies run wild as you decide just who you're riding during this amazing fun and effective self-play!

Did you know they make vibrating Ben Wa balls? Insert a set of these before you vacuum, fill the dishwasher, or even walk the dog. Just don't go too far from home because you're probably not going to last that long!

Peak-a-*Vous*

One of the best ways to ensure intense and powerful orgasms is to get almost all the way there—and then pull back. Then get almost all the way there—and then pull back, again and again.

For this self-pleasuring exercise, you'll need a bullet, the strongest one you can find, and preferably with variable speeds. Take the bullet and start getting yourself all worked up as you count to ten. Then stop, and count to ten again. Then go at it again and again, repeating until you're done.

HOT *lovin'*

Temperature can play a role in bringing on climax, and some women find that turning up the heat on their hot spot not only brings on a faster orgasm, but a more powerful one. Here's a technique that's been known to work wonders. You'll need a warm washcloth (heated in the dryer a few minutes is fine) and one of those black rocks a masseuse uses during a hot stone massage (see Resources).

Place the cloth over your vulva, and place the hot stone on the top of your clitoris, balancing it there with your knees bent and spread to either side. Meditate now for as long as you can, all the while imagining that your heart is beating in your clit. It's amazing when it happens. You know how sometimes after an intense cardio workout, your heart beats so fast and so strong you can feel it in other places? It is truly possible to feel it and move the rock with the beating of your heart. It may take a few tries, but you can actually bring an orgasm on this way (I've done it, and so have clients and friends), by focusing on the heat and channeling all your sexual energy to this one very hot spot.

RELAX *and* REFLECT

Pleasuring yourself in front of a mirror is a great way to gauge what works for you. You may not be able to finish this way, but at least try and start out before you lie back and let the magic happen.

As you pleasure yourself, watch what happens to your body. What do you notice? Do your nipples harden and change color? What about between your legs. Does the color down there change the more excited you get? Afterward, you may want to jot down a few notes about what you learned—maybe even start an orgasm journal so you can track and then study later all the things that got you going. Hey, why not?

nipplegasm

Lots of women swear by their nipples as orgasm aids—and some can even have orgasms just through nipple play. The trick is to build a mental connection between nipple play and orgasming the traditional way. The next time you're stimulating yourself, shift back and forth between your clitoris and your nipples. As your orgasm builds, you'll be training your body and mind to make the association between nipple play and sweet release. But this is not just an "in your head" kind of thing. The increased blood flow to your nipples means increased sensation, which will, in time, lead to more nerve growth. Imagine that! Now you might not get there right away, but you will eventually. And just think of how good it's going to feel to try—and then see if you can create these associations in some of your other parts.

"Nipple Nibblers" is a cream made for nipple stimulation, and it makes your skin tingle. Place a small dab of it down below before you self-stimulate and get ready for the earth to shake! (See Resources.)

UNDERWATER *extravaganza*

Self-pleasuring in the bathtub can be ultrarelaxing, especially if you spread your legs under the faucet as you fill the tub. A scrub brush creates a pleasant sensation when used gently over your hot spot, perhaps also under running water, and a loofah or even a pair of exfoliating gloves are also filled with wonderfully titillating possibilities. They do also make plenty of water-resistant and waterproof vibes now, like the the Body Spa Vibrating Sponge, which has a tiny waterproof vibe in its center—perfect for a shower quickie!

An adjustable showerhead with variable water pulses is a treat; one you can pull off the wall and actually control, positioning the stream of water in just the right way, is a gift from the gods! It's a small investment to make when you consider all the delectable dividends of pleasure this device is sure to deliver.

While it's not marketed as a sex toy, a jelly scrubber makes for an awesome water toy. How do you use it? Remember in the 1980s when DJs used to make scratching noises with records? That's the motion to go for here. Turn on the water, let the warm rush pour all over you, and get ready for your own rush to begin!

IN *dreams* . . .

Studies have shown that 37 percent of women have experienced orgasms during sleep. Amazing, yes, but it makes sense when you think about it. While you're asleep, your conscious mind is shut off, and that means no stresses about paying bills or job strife—or even any of those pesky inhibitions. While we can't really control our dreams, sometimes we can guide them, and that's just what we're going to do here.

Here's the really amazing thing about having an orgasm in your sleep: They don't require any kind of physical stimulation. It's possible to dream you're having an orgasm—and have an orgasm. How cool is that?

How can you have one? There are no guarantees—we really can't control what we dream. But here's something you can try: Before bed, focus on a sexy scenario. It could be one you read in romance novel, or saw in an adult movie—or even one you just made up in your own delightfully dirty mind. As you drift off to sleep, put yourself in the book or the movie and visualize yourself as the character enjoying the most intense and electrifying pleasure. I've been successful trying this out—see if you can have a dreamgasm too.

> Find an adult DVD where the actors are very "vocal" and turn it on before you masturbate. Don't watch—keep your eyes closed and listen as you pleasure yourself and imagine yourself right there in the action. Ooo la la!

OUT OF BODY *O*

Janet, age forty-three, has been married to Ed for nearly eighteen years. She wrote to me for one of my columns that Ed is a medical supplies salesman and is on the road more often than he's home. This has pretty much been the case for most of their marriage. "I like sex, a lot, and I spend a lot of time thinking about it. Also, because Ed is away a lot, I end up taking care of a lot of my own needs sexually. I would never take on a lover—I really do love my husband with all my heart and I really do only want to have sex with him. But sometimes I like to fantasize about other men. I know some of these men. There's the UPS guy who comes around regularly, and the college student that delivers pizza. I also can't watch a movie with Benecio del Toro or Clive Owen in it and not get all hot and bothered. In fact, I have a fantasy that's so incredibly hot involving both Clive and Benecio, I have actually had an orgasm without even touching myself. Does this seem crazy? Are other women able to climax like this—only using their imaginations?"

In the book *The Science of Orgasm*, the authors state that "there are documented cases of women who claim they can experience orgasm just by thinking—without physical stimulation. Their bodily reactions of doubling heart rate, blood pressure, pupil diameter and pain threshold bear out their claim." As I touched on in the last chapter, you can indeed have an orgasm without touching yourself. It takes a lot of focus and concentration, but if you really get your mind off the things that are distracting you, and focus that mind energy into thinking yourself into having O's, you're in for a real treat!

To get yourself in the right frame of mind, take some time every single day to imagine yourself having an orgasm without touching yourself. Imagine that you're being touched in the most perfect way and everything feels wonderful and warm and tingly. You could imagine your lover going down on you, the feel of his warm tongue, his hot breath. The steady rhythmic pulsing of this special kind of kiss . . . You could imagine a scenario in which many different lovers are lined up and ready to please you. Really, it's all up to you and what kinds of fantasies get you going. Here are a few suggestions:

- Fantasize about being with another woman. Many women have this fantasy and it doesn't mean you are a lesbian or even bi. It's about stepping outside the "norm" in your life and exploring something new.
- Fantasize about being with your favorite vampire (I like Bill Compton from *True Blood*) or werewolf or zombie—whatever you're into.
- Fantasize about being with your favorite actor or singer. Male or female, there has to be at least one specimen from the celebrity world you wouldn't mind moving the earth with.
- Does a man in uniform light your fire?
- What about a fireman coming to save you from a burning building?
- A postal worker with a special delivery he needs to deliver with great urgency?
- A pilot who wants to fly your friendly skies?
- How about a businessman?
- A banker in a suit that cost more than your car?
- A college professor in tweed ready to open your mind to all kinds of sexy learning?
- A scientist in a lab coat who's "just this close" to discovering the best pleasuring technique there imaginable and wants to experiment on you? Whatever gets you going!

Again, a great time to do this exercise is right before you go to bed. Not only will the O help you sleep, you'll also have cleared your mind of all of its worries and stresses to get the focus you need for the "Out-of-Body O"—and that means sleeping better!

NOW *you* KNOW

Having great orgasms starts with *you*. Now you're ready to show your partner how to share the pleasure with you. The rest of the book will provide tips and techniques to help him help you get what you need, so be sure to share all "the good parts" with him!

CHAPTER 6

TOUCH ME,
lick ME

"Well, she works hard all day. She's good at her job, why should you care how she unwinds? I mean you like to bake all night, others like to drink, others like an occasional screaming orgasm."
—DR. CRISTINA YANG (SANDRA OH), *GRAY'S ANATOMY*

By now you should have a pretty good, uh, handle on what gets you going and keeps you going, and now it's time to share all you've learned about yourself and your body, your sweet spots, your hot spots, and your *not* spots with that special someone in your life. In this chapter, you'll find tons of surefire manual techniques you can teach your lover to master—with his fingers, hands, toys, and more—as well as oral sex techniques that will leave you sweating, shaking, and full of all kinds of sweet sensations.

Now how you decide to share this information is up to you. You could hand him this book with the most appealing sections highlighted for him to go and study on his own. You could take a more hands-on approach, providing a visual aid as he reads aloud. Whatever you decide, have fun. Connect and communicate and just enjoy the "being together"; when you have those elements in place, the O will be easy. So why not take a cue from Dr. Yang and have yourself a good screaming orgasm tonight!

I CAN'T *do* THAT!

Now that you're an expert on your sexual self, thanks to the lessons in the last chapter, you have so much to share with your partner! Gone are the days of fumbling around in frustration, replaced now by all the glorious sensations touching you just right are going to bring.

So, with all you learned about yourself in the last chapter, it's time to show your lover how you want to be touched. What's your favorite technique from the previous chapter? Which maneuver moved the earth for you? If you don't know right off the bat, take a minute to flip back and reflect. Take more than a minute if you need to. You're about to open the floodgates here, and once you take this step, it's going to be bliss all the way, baby.

Are you nervous? That's okay! Everyone's nervous about doing this. It's a very vulnerable place to be, and especially if you have some insecurity from the past, most everyone feels a little embarrassed and even a little silly. But you have to let that go. You have to trust your partner, and you have to know that all your "audience" wants from you here is your supreme pleasure—and a guide to giving it to you.

So if you need to disguise yourself a little bit to loosen up, that's okay. There's no harm in that. The first time I ever did this for a lover, I wore sunglasses and a wig! I'm not saying you should do that, but there may be some props that might make you feel more comfortable.

The second time I did this, I agreed to take off the sunglasses and wig but insisted that the lights be off. He gently reminded me if the lights were off, he wouldn't be able to see anything and that might ruin the point of it all. Reluctantly, I agreed, but I then insisted the lights be very dim—too dim for him to see, so he suggested candlelight (romantic and useful) and I agreed to that. And this time, even without my "disguise" I felt more and more relaxed.

By the third time, I was okay without a disguise and with the lights on. I had had a glass of wine and I was very relaxed. I trusted him, I was comfortable, and it was a beautiful experience—especially when he was able to then repeat for me everything I had shown him the next time. (And after that, nothing else was ever needed to get me into "the zone.")

Remember if you feel uncomfortable about all this at first, you're not alone. Very few women hit the ground running when it comes to self-pleasuring in front of their partners. But trust me when I tell you: Your male partners want you to do it—and often. They want to learn it more than baseball scores. Well, for the most part maybe.

I had a male client, I'll call him George, whose wife never had an orgasm with him, and he was starting to get worried that she was going to start cheating on him, and soon, if he didn't figure out how to make it work.

"Renee is so beautiful," he told me. "We have such a great relationship in so many other ways. There's just something about this that we can't make work."

I was suspicious that a couple that connected on so many levels couldn't make this part work. I felt that George needed to ask Renee a very important question. "Are you sure she's had orgasms before with other men—men in her past?"

"I don't know," he said. "I just thought it was me who wasn't able to do it for her."

"I know it's not an easy conversation to have," I told him, "but I think you should start by finding out if she's ever had orgasms with other lovers before—and for two reasons. One, if she has, you can open a discussion on things you can do to her that she may have worked for her in the past. And two, and more important I think: If she's never had an orgasm with another lover, you can open that door together."

"How can I do that?"

"Has she had orgasms through self-pleasuring before?"

He was quiet for a minute. "Yes."

"Then she can show you how."

So George went home and had "the talk" with Renee, and he was relieved to learn that it hadn't just been with him that she struggled to climax. He was also pretty excited because now it would be him who could give his wife the pleasure he so wanted to give her and he believed she so deserved.

I advised George on how to make Renee comfortable pleasuring herself for him, and while she was a little resistant at first, she finally allowed herself to relax into it. After years of getting to know herself and bringing herself to orgasm through self-pleasuring, she finally had the comfort level she needed to share this information with her husband—though not completely and not right away.

Renee said it was too difficult to verbally express herself this way, so she wrote down a play by play on how she gave herself an orgasm and sent it to him in an e-mail. His assignment that day was to study her notes and, that evening, follow her direction and see if he could bring her to orgasm this way. He did accomplish it by the fourth try, and they've now gotten so good at it, they're working on how to have an orgasm during sexual intercourse.

Remember: Create your comfort zone, build your connection, and test out the waters a few times. You'll see it will soon all become very natural.

SHOW AND *tell*

Now that you've made a commitment to melt away those inhibitions and you've given yourself a comfort zone in which to do so, the show can begin. Chose a technique from the last chapter and get ready to showcase it. For the purposes of this book, I'm going to take the "Stimulation with Penetration" and walk you through how you can *show and tell* it through for your partner.

Lie down on your bed on your back, or sit in a chair with your legs spread out and hanging over the arms, or lie down on your tummy if you like the added pressure of lying down on your sexy parts. Have plenty of lube at the ready and get yourself nice and slippery as you tell your partner:

"I like it in this position because . . ."

As you lube up your parts, tell him why:

"I like the way this makes me feel all soft and slick down there," or "When my nipples are lubed, it give me extra sensation."

Whatever works for you.

Now take a deep breath and get yourself going. Stimulate your clit or the surrounding area—or both. Talk about the strokes you're taking:

"I like to stroke myself very gently, very lightly at first."

"I don't touch my clit right away. I like to stimulate the left (or right) side first. It's very sensitive."

"I like to tease myself a little first. I get too excited and overwhelmed if I get too much into it right away."

In this case, we're using penetration, so while you're stimulating with one hand, take the other and bring it to your mouth. Lick your fingers and get them extra wet. Tell your lover something to the effect of "I love the warm sensation I get down there when I touch myself after I wet my fingers with my mouth."

As you continue to stimulate yourself with one hand, take the now newly moistened hand and slip your fingers into the orifice of your choice. (Take care if it's your anus you choose that you are very lubed already and that you don't stick your fingers back into your mouth without washing your hands first.) As you penetrate, tell him about the strokes you are taking:

"I like it very slow and smooth at first."

Or:

"By this point I'm so crazed and ready, that I like to penetrate myself fast and furious while I get more intense on the motion with my other hand."

You may also choose to penetrate yourself with a sex toy, and we'll talk more about those options as we get deeper into this chapter. But whether you use your hand or a sex toy, be sure to use plenty of lube; and if you've used either one anally, don't place your hand or toy in any other openings until your hand or the toy is washed with warm water and soap.

Above all, remember that what I've given you here is not a script. These are guidelines for things to say and simple ways to express them. You have to write your own script depending on what feels right for you! It's all about what feels good.

all IN!

How empowered are you feeling right now? Empowered enough to have your partner play along? Then tell him to grab some lube and whatever else you chose and invite him to hop on up!

Tell your partner that you are going to talk him through doing everything you just taught him. Try to resist touching yourself; see how powerfully you can convey your message simply through your words, your breathing, your moans, and even your body language.

Is your partner doing what you want him to? Don't get frustrated or annoyed. Gently remind him "Less pressure" or "Circles now, not back and forth," or "That's too many fingers inside me right now, let's get more warmed up first." When he's doing it right, tell him. "That feels great" or "That feels wonderful" will communicate your message to him simply and wonderfully. He wants to do this right. He wants to make you feel good. The more encouragement you give him when he's doing what he's supposed to do, the better he's going to get.

Remember: A man does not naturally know what makes you feel good because what makes him feel good is so different. You've given a hand-job to a man before. You know he likes it tight, rough, fast. He needs to be reminded that you are built differently than he is.

And don't be afraid to amp up the noise! If you like what he's doing, moan loud. Breathe into it. Let your breathing and your sounds carry you away. Two words that pop into my head as you're getting close to climax are *surrender* and *relax*. When he's gotten his "training" down, surrender yourself to his touch and all the wonderful sensations you are beginning to feel. And relax and let that orgasm take you. Some of the best orgasms I've ever had have been from hand stimulation alone. How about you?

fore-FOREPLAY

Gentlemen, repeat after me: A woman's main sex organs are not her genitals. One more time: A woman's main sex organs are not her genitals. They are her mind and her soul and her skin. You should never make a beeline for the lady parts like you're trying to hit a target and there's some button you can press for instant satisfaction. It doesn't exist on her and it will only leave the two of you feeling frustrated and unfulfilled.

If you launch right into the business of genital stimulation without so much as a cuddle, kiss, snuggle, or kind word, you're going to be spending a lot of time exhausting yourself rubbing and licking as you try to arouse her. And why would you do that when you could accomplish the same feat in minutes—even seconds—by taking the time to pleasure those top two organs first?

Did you know that foreplay goes back a lot further than a kiss or a grazing of the nipples or a fondling of other lady parts? Foreplay can start with a look or an innocent touch—and it can also build with a less-innocent touch, like a sexy massage.

Not only does the relaxation aspect of this kind of massage help clear all the clutter out of her brain and start her really focusing on her body, but the sensation of you touching her all over also means she'll be ready to explode when you finally touch her in an overtly sexual way. Here's a massage technique from *A Little Bit Kinky* that readers have written in and confirmed that it has launched their lovers well on their way to mind-blowing passion.

Make sure she's in a comfy space—on the couch, on the bed, on a soft rug by the fireplace—and ask her to undress. Light a candle and make sure to have the massage oils at the ready.

Relax her shoulders by kneading them on each side of her shoulder blades. Ask for her input. Does she want more pressure? Does she want less?

Work down to her lower back, making small circular motions with your thumbs. When you get to her buns, rub the inside of your forearm in large circular motions on her rear, one cheek at a time. This is what I like to call bun bliss.

Instruct her to roll over and kneel by her left side. Gently lift her arm, placing her elbow in your palm. With a light touch from your fingertips, stroke the inside area of her arm. Then take your thumbs and work on the forearms by alternating, pressing in until you get to the hands and knead the hand with your thumbs, alternating. Interlace her fingers with yours and pull back on her palm with your hand, gently now. Give her hand a soft, gentle kiss and do the other side.

Rub her legs with long strokes using the palms of your hands. Alternate between them and push your strokes toward her heart.

Move down to her feet. Place a pillow under her knees as she's lying face up and with your flat open palms, massage the entire foot, slowly and evenly. Move your thumbs in mini circles then alternate pressing and kneading with your thumbs. (Did you know that the feet are a major erogenous zone?)

Last, massage her scalp. Take the earlobes in between your thumb and index fingers and rub in little circles, then slide your palms on either side of her head, gently lifting the roots of her hair upward. Lightly scratch her head all over; then with your fingertips, lightly massage her temples. Lightly massage her whole head in big circles with your fingertips and finish with the earlobe massage.

After a massage as intense as this, most women will be revved up and ready to go. But don't be too annoyed if you actually relax her so much she falls asleep. She'll make it up to you.

quick fix } TINGLING WITH DESIRE

Nympho's Desire is an enriched arousal cream that heightens erogenous zone sensitivity and enhances sexual response. I swear by it! Dab a little dollop around her clitoris, and use more as needed. It will begin to tingle her and feel hot. Keep massaging around her vaginal area with your fingers as you would massage any other part of the body, *but don't use inside her.* As her heat intensifies, so will her orgasm, and she will go insane with lust!

LISTEN *up*, GUYS!

Now that you've been able to focus on other parts of your lady, let's get into the nitty-gritty of really *hand*-ling her. Of course, it's a thrill to be able to bring your woman to the brink and beyond with some carefully crafted maneuverings of your manly fingers, but it's definitely not a skill you're born with. It takes practice—and plenty of it. It takes listening and feeling things out (while you're feeling them up). Here are some good pointers for you:

Wash your hands and trim your nails.

The vulva and all its parts is actually quite delicate and there's nothing more unpleasant than a fissure caused by a jagged fingernail—unless it's a urinary tract or bladder infection caused by dirty hands and fingers. Keep it clean and smooth, please!

Remove jewelry.

By this I don't mean a simple wedding band. But if you're a rock star type who likes to wear lots of complicated rings and things, take them off. All that hardware can become quite uncomfortable when you're playing with her "software."

Take it slow.

There is no place in the world you'd rather be right now and no place more important you need to rush to get to. Take your time with her. The less you rush, the faster you'll get her there—trust me!

Lube it up.

Remember: Clean and smooth. Don't force your fingers inside her if she isn't ready to accept them. Massage around the area and moisten your fingers before using them—with your mouth or hers!

Change it up.

Don't just massage in circles and don't just go back and forth. The motion needs to change or it will get as redundant for her as it may start getting for you.

Touch her—everywhere.

And not just where it seems obvious, like her breasts and shoulders. A lot of women respond quite favorably to having their tummies rubbed while you stimulate them. Makes sense as it's another way to get all the blood flowing right to where you want it! With a light touch, and in a clockwise motion, graze her tummy first with your fingertips and escalate to your palms. Focus on the area right below the belly button and right above her pubic hair—but do not touch the pubic region. Are you able to scratch or rub her tummy as you manually stimulate her with your other hand or orally pleasure her? Try it—and maybe she can even lend a hand. It will bring her the orgasm of her life.

Play some relaxing music in the background.

Not only will the music soothe her, it will block out the other distractions that may be happening close by, like a too-loud TV in the family room or the neighbors arguing with their bedroom window open again.

Say her name and compliment her.

Tell her how you feel about her and make her feel she's the only person in the universe for that moment. For example: "Lisa, you look so beautiful." "Arianna, I'm so turned on by you."

Kiss her.

Absolutely do not forget to kiss her while you're stimulating her manually. Kiss her neck and her chest, her tummy and her shoulders, and, most importantly, her mouth. Kick up the intensity with intimacy. A deep, sensuous kiss at the moment of climax will ensure a deep, sensuous orgasm!

SENSITIVE PLACES,
wonderful THINGS

The clitoral head is indeed the most sensitive part of the clitoris, but it can become over stimulated very quickly and easily. So unless you know for certain that your lover likes and needs plenty of direct clitoral stimulation to get her going, I recommend taking long breaks away from it. Stimulate by all means, but then turn your attention to something else and come back. And then turn your attention to another part of her, like her nipples or her knees, and then come back to stimulating her clit.

Also, you may already know that one side of her clitoris is more sensitive than the other. That's a great thing to know about your lover, but it also doesn't mean that's the only side you and your partner need to focus on all the time. A little teasing by stimulating the other side—and coming oh so close to grazing the sensitive part—will go a long way in prolonging ecstasy.

And I can't seem to say this enough: It's not just about the clit! Stimulate the outer labia and the inner labia. The clitoris extends underneath the surface of the inner labia. Take your well-lubed index finger and middle finger and massage up and down her labia then gently place these two fingers at the top entrance to her vagina and lightly, and gently, rub back and forth on that area. Now, do it all over again and again and again. Do the above, but this time add your second hand to gently spread open her labia and trace ovals around the inside of her inner labia.

Here's another neat trick that involves her whole nether region: Apply lots of lube both to your hand and to her vulva. Now straighten your hand, and with the pinky side, rub gently against each side of her inner labia in a sawing motion. Then make a V with the index finger and middle finger on the same hand, and glide up and down on each side of her clitoris. Last, but not least, lube your palm and place it just under the clitoris as you massage the entirety of the vagina in big circles to the right for ten and then to the left for ten, and repeat until she lets you know it's time.

Massage her body and follow your movements with light tongue strokes. Go over her entire body like this, massaging and licking every inch of her—but not her vaginal region, at least not yet. Get her all tingly with desire. Now manually stimulate her clitoris—with the head of your penis. Pretend the tip of your penis is an extension of your finger and gently make eight circles around the clitoris to the right, then eight to the left. Pulse upward underneath the clitoris eight times then push just the tip of your penis in her vagina. Repeat this over and over again, each time giving her just a little more of your penis. The more you prolong her delicious "agony," the more the sexual tension will build in her and the more explosive her orgasm will be.

And don't forget about her other "*spots*." Take your hand and curve it into a C. Lube your thumb and gently insert it into her vagina. Now with your hand curved like a hook over her pubic bone, rock it back and forth, using your palm to stimulate her clitoris while your thumb stimulates her G-spot and the inside of your hand stimulates her U-spot. (The U-spot is a sensitive area between the vagina and the urethra that in fairly recent studies has shown to be a hot button of orgasmic potential when stimulated by hand, tongue, or the tip of a penis.) To heighten her pleasure past her wildest expectation, seal it now with a kiss. In other words, go down on her, gently dabbing at her clitoris while you continue the rocking motion. Mastering this technique alone will make you a total sex god in her eyes.

Here are some other variations she may enjoy:

• Lightly flicker your finger back and forth across the head of her clitoris.

- Gently tap the head of the clitoris.
- Rest a finger inside her vagina while you do the above.
- Thrust two fingers gently inside and out while you do the above.
- Thrust two fingers gently along the front wall of the vagina where the G-spot is (and ask her to guide you to her G-spot if you're having trouble locating it).
- Gently massage the bottom wall of the vagina with two fingers while applying medium pressure.
- Flatten your hand and massage the vulva in big circles to the right and then to the left.

How about giving your lover a double orgasm? When you manually stimulate your partner, use a soft, slow touch. Move your index finger around and around her clitoris in light circles. When you get to ten, lightly skim the top of the clitoris and reverse the direction for ten more circles. As her excitement builds, slowly glide the index finger of your free hand into her vagina, focus on rubbing the tip of your finger on the upper front wall of her vagina. The desired result is a double orgasm (clitoral and G-spot).

toygasm!

Arthur was another male client of mine who came to see me at the behest of his wife, Michelle. Both in their late forties, Arthur and Michelle had been married for more than twenty years, and Michelle was looking to spice things up between them when she brought a Rabbit vibe into bed with them. "Arthur's a really conservative guy," she told me on the phone while I waited for Arthur to arrive for his appointment. "I think it really freaked him out," she said. "I should have thought it through. I should have talked it over with him first instead of just springing it on him! I mean, the guy won't even let you call him anything but Arthur!"

I assured Michelle that Arthur would be in good hands just as my buzzer rang. I hung up with her and greeted Arthur, who, in his buttoned-up Oxford shirt and pressed pants was exactly as I imagined he would look on a Saturday morning.

"I'm only here for my wife," he started defensively. "I mean, for us both actually. I don't think she's satisfied anymore and it's gotten me worried sick."

"Have a seat, Artie, and we'll talk," I baited.

"It's Arthur," he corrected.

"Of course," I smiled. "So tell me the problem."

He hesitated and he started to turn bright red. "The other night . . ." he began, but left off there.

"This is about the vibrator?" I asked.

"Uh yeah," he said, not looking at me.

"You're not sure why she—"

"Why does she need that thing!" He nearly jumped out of his seat. "Do you mean to tell me that after twenty-some-odd years together, she's just telling me now that I don't do it for her? That she needs this thing, this device, instead of me?"

I motioned for him to sit down again. "On the contrary," I told him. "Your wife is delighted with you sexually. She's so excited to be with you sexually, in fact, all she wants to do is to expand each of your sexual horizons together. This is actually a really good thing."

"It is?"

"It definitely is."

Here's the thing: A lot of guys get freaked out by sex toys. But they shouldn't. In many ways, sex toys are a girl's best friend—and they can be a guy's as well. There is nothing to fear when it comes to sex toys. They are not meant to replace you; they are meant to enhance what you can do with your lover to bring her pleasure. Think of a vibrator as a third hand or another appendage at the ready—just always remember to use plenty of lube. The possibilities are limited only by your imagination and inhibitions.

Here are some ideas:

· Rest a vibrator on the area around your lover's clit as you kiss and stroke her nipples and breasts.
· Place a washcloth over her vulva. Rest a vibrating vibrator on top and see what happens.
· Insert a vibrator into her vagina as you massage her vulva and clit.
· Insert a vibrator into her anus, as you insert a finger into her vagina, and massage her clit with your other hand.
· Insert a vibrator into her vagina and go down on her at the same time.
· Experiment with a vibrator on her nipples, behind her knees, maybe even to tickle those toes.
· Buy a massage mitt, drop a vibrating bullet into it, and voila! A vibrating hand for full body massages!

Not all sex toys are created for that purpose, however. Consider something as innocent as a cucumber or perhaps squash. You don't have to look far to realize that your refrigerator and even your entire kitchen holds a lot of sexy toys and lube too. If you plan on playing with fruit or vegetables though, just be sure you always use a condom and lots of lube before inserting them anywhere.

I had a client who was quite "creative" in the kitchen, meaning she really enjoyed sex play with food. Especially long, firm foods. At first it kind of freaked her man out, but when they came to me together and I gave this kind of play the "okay," it became clear that all he was looking for was permission. While what she liked may have been a bit offbeat, it wasn't totally deviant.

So he decided to give in. Later, they described an evening of organic erotica to me, telling me that they had gone to the organic grocery store to shop for dinner one night. She decided to turn the evening into an erotic date night, and she then shopped for items she thought would be good for sex play—and also make for great "toys." Their groceries consisted of honey, chocolate syrup, different-sized cucumbers, squashes, zucchini, apples, and carrots, tortillas, and hot sauce.

They played with the phallic vegetables first. Slipping condoms around the cucumbers, squashes, zucchini, and carrots, and using a liberal amount of lube each time, they experimented with different lengths and widths, and they discovered what sizes were the most satisfying (and not always the biggest ones!) for her. Later, they chopped up their leftover "sex toys" and turned them into veggie tacos. For dessert they fed each other apple slices with honey and chocolate syrup.

In addition to making your skin feel all slippery and sexy, massage oils actually "spread out" sensation when you're using a vibrator. The oil acts as a conduit for the vibrations—much in the same way electricity travels through water.

YOUR *toy* CLOSET

Sex toys are orgasm machines—literally. There are so many possibilities, both in variety and in potency. From small vibes to Realistics and butt plugs, there really is something for everyone. Here's a breakdown of sex toys I created for *A Little Bit Kinky* and have expanded on. You might consider having a few in your carnal closet. And while there are sex toys specifically designed for women and for men, as far as I'm concerned, most can be used to pleasure both—and in so many wonderful ways.

Bullets and **Eggs** are excellent for clitoral stimulation. "Bnaughty" is waterproof, has multiple speeds, and is my personal favorite bullet. Cyberflicker is my favorite egg.

The Pink Pop vibrating love bullet is also one of my faves for learning how to orgasm, and it's great to use during sex to orgasm during the actual act.

My First Vibe and **Slimline** are basic cylindrical vibes. Many first timers start here and use it for vaginal and anal stimulation and penetration. The sizes vary, and when possible, always get the option for variable speed vibration.

Realistic looks like a penis and is good for penetration and fantasy.

The Jolie: Intense Clitoral Pleasure is 100 percent waterproof (so it can be used in the bathtub) and compact, but it packs a punch!

The **Libertie** has three speeds and is excellent for G-spot stimulation.

The **Ideal** is similar to the Hitachi Magic Wand (see page 146) but it's smaller—which means more flexibility in terms of sex positions.

Mini massagers like the **Pocket Rocket** are great for clitoral stimulation and small enough to fit in your purse.

Crystal Wand, Nubby G Vibe, G-Whiz are all excellent G-spot stimulators.

Fantasy Fingers, Finger Fun, Fukuoku 9000 are my favorite finger vibes.

The **Laya Spot** works great for clitoral stimulation.

SaSi Vibrator is my latest discovery—and it's amazing! Contoured and smooth, it vibrates softly, and the movement type, speed, and vibration are all adjustable. But that's not the best part. SaSi has "Sensual Intelligence," which means you can program it to remember your favorite speed and movement.

The **Rock Chick** is a U-shaped toy with a hooked end for G-spot stimulation and a wider, ridged end for clitoral and labia stimulation. You use it by rocking, and rocking the toy forward and back nudges the G-spot and rubs the clitoris at the same time.

Tongue Joy is a wonderful, vibrating toy that fastens to your tongue for some serious oral pleasure—for you and her.

Turbo Bullet is a small vibe—small enough that it fits in your mouth. Pull it out while you're going down on your partner. Now turn it on and slip it into your mouth, rolling it around with your tongue. Now, as you pleasure her, wherever your tongue goes, the toy follows. Just be very careful not to choke!

Alia by Lelo is a pricey but gorgeous waterproof clitoral stimulator.

Selene Clitoral & Nipple Suction by Dr. Berman is great for increasing blood flow and your chances of orgasm.

NEA is another amazing clitoral massager I really enjoy using.

The **Ina, Rabbit Habit, and Rosebud** are all toys that stimulate both the clitoris and the G-spot.

The **Little Flirt** is a great butt plug for beginners, and the **B-Bomb** is one that vibrates. (Let's face it: women's G-spots are easily stimulated indirectly through anal play.)

naughty NIPPLES

Women are more aroused by breast and nipple stimulation than men during lovemaking, according to the first ever evidence-based research, published in the May 2006 issue of *The Journal of Sexual Medicine*. And there are so many ways to arouse them, but don't manhandle the breasts. Instead, use the light touch of the tip of your tongue or blow on them. Here are some techniques for nipple stimulation that have been known to drive women wild. As you experiment, encourage her to rate each experience from one to ten—with ten being superfantastic and one being "never, never again."

- Treat her to a breast massage with a sweet-smelling massage oil.
- Rub your hands together for warmth and then touch her breasts.
- Massage around and around the breasts, getting to the nipples last.
- Draw circles around her breasts with your index finger and then lightly touch her nipples.
- Dab some Nipple Nibblers on her nipples.
- Lick her nipples and then blow on them. Suck them and kiss them.
- Use your eyelashes and give her nipples butterfly kisses.
- Vibrate a toy on her breasts and nipples.
- If you dare, try some nipple clamps or vibrating nipple clamps!

I had a client who wanted to become more nipple sensitive. She had never really been into her boobs before because she always felt they were too small. I told her there was no such thing as breasts that were too small! So we needed to work to get her more interested in them.

Several nights a week, I encouraged her to read an erotic short story before going to bed. While she was reading or after, I told her she was to lie in bed and massage her breasts and fantasize about what she had read. The idea here was to help make herself feel good via breast-and-nipple stimulation alone. I told her it was okay if she wanted to use oils or toys, but she was restricted to breast-and-nipple stimulation only. I told her that she could also have her husband join in and they could even have intercourse, but there could be no other foreplay until the fourth week of the program.

Then, after four weeks, I told her it was okay now for her hubby to stimulate her breasts and nipples and also her clitoris. She needed to tell him that what he had to do was to go back and forth from stimulating her clitoris to her breasts and nipples several times and then do all at the same time until she had an orgasm.

She said she began feeling the orgasms in her breasts even though they were generating from her clitoris. We rewired and tied it all in. The body is amazing that way!

oral PLEASURES

I did a survey years ago for women and how they had their best orgasms, and the hands-down winner was through oral sex. And then in another survey, I learned that the sexual pleasuring women are least likely to ask for is . . . wait for it . . . *oral*. For real! So how can that be?

Here's another thing I learned: Many women do not feel comfortable asking for and even receiving pleasure orally. Some women said they worried about the way they tasted or smelled down there. Others were more concerned with how they looked—that they weren't that comfortable with their partner seeing their vulva so up close and personal.

I say there is no reason whatsoever you shouldn't ask for and receive tons of oral pleasure! First of all, your guy really likes what you look like down there. Nature has designed you perfectly to appeal to his sense of aesthetics in this realm. If he thinks your vulva is ugly, he might not be straight. And guess what? They're also programmed to be drawn to the scent of "down there," yes, just like dogs. Now I'm not saying never clean yourself. And if it makes you more comfortable to wipe down with a warm soapy washcloth or even take a shower beforehand, there's certainly no harm in that. All I'm saying is that it doesn't matter to him as much as it matters to you. In fact, many men do enjoy the *au naturel* approach. But again, if it makes you feel better to be clean, there's certainly no harm in it!

VICTORIA'S *secret*

Victoria, age twenty-three, has never been comfortable receiving oral sex, but her boyfriend Mike was so into giving it, she generally just gave in.

"I don't know what the appeal is," she told me. "He wants to go down on me all the time—even in the morning before I've been able to take a shower. It can be a little horrifying, honestly. I mean, especially if we had sex the night before and I haven't cleaned any of that away yet!"

I asked her if she enjoyed it on any level.

"Well, sure," she said. "I guess. I mean, it feels really good at first. Really warm and wet. But then my mind wanders. What if I look ugly down there? What if I smell terrible but he's just being nice about everything? Then I can't relax anymore thinking about these things and I only want it all to be over!"

"Does he act like he wants it to be over?"

"Well no," she said. "But again, I think this is just because he's trying to be nice, you know?"

I tried to explain to her that if it was so unpleasant for him he probably wouldn't pursue it as aggressively as he does, and she started to agree with me but then let herself go back into her own head again. "It always takes me so long to come, and then I feel really bad about it because it's got to be exhausting and boring for him."

I told her that the first thing she needed to do was to stop projecting, but I also let her know that her fears and her feelings were actually quite common—and especially for someone her age. But I also let her know that a life without oral was probably not going to be as much fun as it could be for her, and I convinced her to listen and learn about how to have an enjoyable, stress-free orgasm this way.

On her own time, I told her to sit in front of a mirror or pick up a hand mirror and examine her vulva. I told her to take a good look and write down for me what she liked and didn't like about it. During our next session, we surfed the Internet together and looked at hundreds of vulvas of other women. After that, she started to feel more comfortable about hers. She had thought hers was ugly and different and deformed, but really it was so similar to many we saw that day that it made her more comfortable. The issue was not more than this.

The next step to tackle was the scent issue. We determined she was most comfortable receiving oral after a bath or shower. I also suggested she take a wet washcloth and simply wipe herself before oral. Then I asked her to ask Mike what some of his favorite scents were. She did and it turns out he didn't like perfume or oils but preferred everything natural.

The last hurdle was the "why" it was taking her so long to orgasm. I instructed her to be more verbal and tell Mike what she likes and how she likes it. When he's on a spot that's getting her there, she needed to tell him so he doesn't switch to some other type of stimulation.

Last but not least, I told her to keep a vibrating bullet nearby. If it was taking too long in her opinion, I told her she was to take the bullet and put it on or near her clitoris while he licked around it and see what happens. All the suggestions worked,and eventually they didn't need to use the toy.

LICK HER HOWSHE *likes* IT

Just as it was with manual stimulation, women do not like the same kinds of stimulation that men do. They are built differently; they respond to sensations differently. If you like rough suction and lots of hand action when she goes down on you, great! But that may not be what she's all about. Here are some pretty safe tips. You need to try these on her and then pay attention to how she responds and what she responds best to if you really want to satisfy her!

Plan for an orgasm.

Make sure everybody is comfortable right from the start—that both you and your partner are both in comfortable positions before you get started.

Start out right.

Be sure to pull back the clitoral hood so the clitoris is exposed and standing to attention.

Lightly at first.

Experiment with the surface of your tongue as you pleasure her. Fold it, flatten it, point it, and swirl it around her clitoris.

Turn up the intensity.

Stiffen your tongue and dip it into her vagina every thirty seconds or so.

Sound it out.

Move your tongue over her clitoris pronouncing tuh-kuh tuh-kuh over and over again. Then gently suck on her clitoris. Then repeat the tuh-kuh-tuh-kuh.

Breathe heavy.

Exhale deeply as you go down on her and let her savor the sensation of your hot breath—which also feels good on the nipples.

Kiss her lovingly.

Kiss her lips down there as you would her lips up there.

bonus ROUND!

The great thing about the mouth is it is such a natural sex toy—it is warm, wet, and soft! The following are some tasty ways your partner can go downtown on you. Please share these with them.

The Kitty Kat

Use your whole tongue to lap up and down her vulva like a cat lapping up a bowl of cream. Up down, up down, up down.

Circle Time

Point your tongue and trace little circles around her clitoris and then bigger circles around the entrance to her vagina.

The Figure Eight

Point your tongue and trace figure eights all over her sexy parts. The top of the eight is around her clitoris, and the bottom is around the lower part of her labia.

The Ice Cream Sandwich

With both hands, press her inner and outer labia together (the cake part) and then lick up and down the length of her lips (the ice cream!).

The Suction Cup

Place your mouth over her clitoris and create suction. This creates a nice vacuum effect, which will in turn increase blood flow into the clitoris making it easier for her to orgasm.

The Tasty Treat

Try any of the above techniques using a flavored lubricant.

The Tingly Trick

Use a product called nipple nibblers on her clit. Just a dab will do. Now lick around the clit and occasionally over it.

The Tongue Vibe

Purchase a vibrating tongue toy and stimulate her with it in all the ways above.

Crazy Combo

Go back and forth stimulating her with your tongue and then with a finger vibe—back and forth, again and again, until she explodes with pleasure!

CAPPUCCINO *dreams*

A female client of mine shared this amazingly sexy scenario with me after her fourth date with the guys she's starting to believe is "the one." Basically, after dinner he talked her into having dessert back at his place. There, he made some frothy, warm cappuccinos and they sat at the coffee table in his living room to drink them. She was wearing a thin dress and a very tiny pair of panties. They had been together before, though not all the way, but she was ready for him. In fact, she had decided that this was going to be "the night," and it looked like he was into it to.

"And then he asked me if I liked the taste of coffee," she blushed. "I took a sip from my mug and told him the cappuccino was great—and then he asked about my 'other lips.' Before I knew what happened, he had taken a big swig from his mug, held it in his mouth, and dove under my dress. Somehow he managed to keep the coffee in his mouth as he pulled the thin string of my G-string out of the way and started to pleasure me with the coffee in his mouth. Talk about hot oral sex!"

The thrill of this technique comes from the warmth of the beverage, and if you're not a coffee drinker, any hot beverage will do. The trick is to keep the liquid in your mouth! Here's a cool (okay, hot) technique I developed and gets raves from clients all the time:

1. Flatten your tongue and lap around and around her clitoris, counterclockwise, for a count of ten. Reverse for another count of ten.

2. Now place your middle and index fingers inside her vagina, applying moderate pressure to the G-spot area. Leave your fingers inside her and don't move them around except to press upward.

3. Lightly suck on her clitoris, placing your whole mouth over it and lightly flicking it with your pointed tongue.

4. Arrange your body so your lips parallel her lips. Pucker your lips and lightly brush your lips to hers back and forth, back and forth, repeat several times then stick your tongue out just enough to poke out from your lips and continue until she reaches her climax.

crossing THE FINISH LINE

As a woman approaches orgasm, she may breathe heavily, moan, or writhe more and more, but this doesn't necessarily mean she wants you to make the stimulation more vigorous. Ask her if she wants you to go faster, slower, or at a steady pace.

After she orgasms, her clitoris will more than likely be really sensitive so she might want you to stop stimulating it or she might want you to keep going for a multiple, but she's the only one who knows so ask her what she wants next. After it's all over, it is nice to embrace your partner and tell her how you feel about her. Hug her, kiss her, and hold her tight! Try not to rush up and off without having at least a little cool down time.

NOW *you* KNOW

Of course, pleasuring to orgasm is something you can do on your own and learn to do really well, but it can also be a lot of fun with a partner. As always, the key is to keep an open mind and to make a commitment to communicate and connect.

Oral and manual stimulation are the main ways women are able to achieve orgasm, but many have climaxed during intercourse as well. There are tricks to this, and they sometimes incorporate the techniques learned in this chapter, but it isn't impossible to orgasm during sex. Now let's find out how!

CHAPTER 7

ASSUME THE POSITIONS

"Seen through the glow of a building orgasm, a woman seems to blaze with angelic glory."
—LARRY NIVEN, AMERICAN SCIENCE-FICTION AUTHOR

Studies show that women are more likely to orgasm with the aid of or simply from oral stimulation than they are through sexual intercourse alone. But no woman on the planet needs a study to tell her that! Let's face facts here: The hardest way for any woman to orgasm is during intercourse. Why? Because we're *not* designed to get climax from an in-and-out motion. The friction of intercourse is what makes a man come. That in-and-out also misses most of our sensitive parts. Of course it feels good in other ways, but the likelihood that any one of us is going to come that way without any other assistance is incredibly rare.

The number of women who climax through sexual intercourse alone is so low it's almost miraculous that it happens at all. Yet, we women really come down on ourselves hard when we can't come that way. We think there's something wrong with us—that we're defective somehow. Crazy when you know how common *not* having an orgasm during intercourse is!

That's just the way it is. That's Nature; you can't change your physiology, and there's no reason why you should. We have options—and even during the act. In this chapter, we'll provide you with detailed descriptions and diagrams of the most orgasmic sexual positions for women to bring you to climax during the act. And not only are we going to look at the sexual positions most likely to produce an orgasm for you, we'll also look at all the wonderful ways you get to "cheat" while getting the penile penetration you crave.

> Keep kissing during sex and you'll maintain a powerful emotional connection while you ride, thrust, and grind—and a more intense orgasm at that!

TAKE *that*, NATURE!

Erin, a thirty-something human resources consultant, came to see me several months ago because she was frustrated with her sex life. "Of course I have orgasms," she said to me sadly (sadly?!), "but I want to start having them, you know, the 'natural' way."

"The natural way?" I asked.

"You know, during sex. I mean, I've gotten really close. Sometimes when my boyfriend and I do it doggie-style, I'm almost there. But then . . . I don't know. I just can't cross the finish line. It's like I'm defective or something."

Part of me wanted to chuckle. Part of me wanted to reach out and shake her. But the biggest part of me was sad about the situation because as I said above, women really do believe that if they can't climax during intercourse, everything else is somehow unnatural. I took a deep breath and exhaled. "What makes you think that having an orgasm during sex is the only 'natural' way to have one?"

She looked at me for a minute and then said, "Well, you never see women in movies needing any 'extra' help."

"Do you believe everything you see in movies?" I asked her.

"I guess not," she replied and looked away. "But I have friends too. Friends who say they can climax during sex."

"Have you ever asked them how—I mean *specifically*, in full uncensored detail, how they manage this?"

"No."

"Good. Because I'm going to tell you now."

I explained to her the design of the vulva, the placement of the clitoris, and angles of penetration. I showed her with a model how nine times out of ten a penis that's attached to a man that has other parts like a torso, can't always achieve the angle that's needed to stimulate a clitoris. "It's just plain physics," I told her, and she began to understand.

My advice to her was to continue practicing in the position that had given her the most positive result: rear entry, or doggie-style. Then I suggested that while she and her boyfriend were going at it, either he should reach around and stimulate her clitoris in the way she would teach him that she liked it or that while he was penetrating her she do it herself.

She came back the next week and said they had tried it, but they just couldn't get it to work. That's also not uncommon. Think of the level of multitasking that one needs to have when neither you nor your partner is in your right frame of mind to concentrate on massage patterns, pressure applied, and that kind of thing. So I gave her another recommendation.

"A vibrator?" she asked, seeming a bit scandalized. "But that's not even a little bit natural!"

I explained to her that Nature made the brain that devised the invention and that even Nature can celebrate being improved upon. She agreed to give it a try.

I recommended the Hitachi Magic Wand (the big daddy of vibes) for her, and that the next time she was having sex with her boyfriend, she was to whip it out and place it on or near her clitoris or even on her lower abdomen. She chose to place it just above her clit and *boom!* She had an orgasm.

I told her that this should be just the beginning of their experimentation and that there were many other things she could try (positions, for instance, that we'll go through in this chapter). But I also assured her that if this was the only way she can have an orgasm during sex, she should celebrate that she found the way. "There is no right or wrong way to have an orgasm during sexual intercourse," I told her.

THE *warm*-UP

All women require at least some level of foreplay before intercourse to ensure that an orgasm will result. Yes, there are a handful of women who can go from 0 to 60 in a minute flat, but most of us need our engines revved a bit before we peak. Men, on the other hand, are not like this. Say the word *sex* to your partner and his "piston" will pop up immediately, fully prepared to probe. So even though you've probably told your lover time and again that you need a little action before the action, you may find yourself having to tell him this again and again. Be patient—he can't help how excited and lucky he feels that beautiful you actually wants to have sex with him!

Remember that foreplay does not have to be overtly sexual. Of course it can be, but it could also be something that starts to put you in the right mood, like a warm bath. Or that awakens your senses, like a full-body massage. Or even something that strips away some of the drudgery of life—like your partner putting the kids to bed! Foreplay is anything that relaxes you and opens you up for getting turned on.

Here's a technique I've recommended to couples where you actually count the levels of arousal from anything he may be doing to you and for you. The scale goes from 1 to 10, with 1 being "Hey, I'm starting to get aroused" and 10 being "Whoa! Bring it home now, baby!" Maybe he's rubbing your shoulders or caressing you. Maybe he's massaging your breasts or stimulating you with his fingers. Maybe he's giving you the tongue-lashing of your life! Try and stop whatever's going on at around 7 and start having intercourse. It's very possible the excitement of the penetration could very well push you over the edge into ecstasy!

My client Frieda wanted desperately to have orgasms during intercourse, but she never could. It was a source of constant frustration for her. I tried to find out from her why the orgasms she had from manual and oral stimulation weren't satisfying her, but she couldn't really explain why. "I just always have this fantasy of myself getting pummeled by this sexy, wonderful man with rippling muscles and a giant you-know-what, and in my fantasy, I climax time after time, just from him being inside of me!"

"That's a pretty good fantasy," I told her.

"I know," she said, with a sly smile.

"But you know, that really is just a fantasy. Right?"

I then went on to explain to her all the orgasmic elements of the human female anatomy, and while there were orgasmic areas aside from the clitoris, this was indeed the "magic button."

"So if I'm not getting any kind of clitoral stimulation, I'm probably not going to come that way."

"Probably not. But you can train yourself to be orgasmic in other places you know," I told her, which we covered back in chapter 4. "You just have to build a powerful association and let your mind convince your body it's possible."

"I'll try anything!" she said.

My favorite kind of client.

I had Frieda practice the excitement scale exercise above with her boyfriend Mark. When she found herself close to 7, a sensation she was getting from his licking and lapping, she pulled him away and encouraged him to enter her. She told me that they began having sex then, but very slow—almost excruciatingly slow.

"I told him to think and move in slow motion," she said.

"Good advice," I told her.

Moving that way may have felt unnatural at first, but it was important for prolonging the ecstasy. "I wanted him so badly I could just scream!" she said.

Frieda told me her arousal level shot through the roof and all she wanted was him inside her bad. Only on her prompting was he permitted to go deeper and faster. Sometimes she would have an orgasm and sometimes she would get close. During the times where it wasn't working, she found that if she switched to being on top after all this excitement it was almost always a sure thing. So don't be afraid to try variations of everything you've learned in this book!

WORKING INTO *it*

Just as men are prone to hone in on you and expect you to be ripe and ready as they are, many of them also start the act of intercourse in much the same way. They slide themselves in and begin to thrust fiercely and madly. You have to stop this! Do you know why? Here's the thing: Most women actually find the first sensation of penetration to be one of the most exciting aspects of sex. In fact, guys, if you take your time and pay attention to the initial entry, you'll see it actually feels really good for both parties. So what's the rush? When your lover thrusts in, have him pull out all the way and then pay attention to the other parts of you, like your neck or your nipples. Then he can come back in again—and then pull out again. Then he can enter you again and leave again. Stop and start; stop and start. Do this for as many times as both of you can withstand, and you may find that you'll both come quickly and powerfully.

GET YOUR HEAD *right*

Sometimes women can be so focused on other things they can't wrap their brains around having an orgasm. And sometimes women are so hyperfocused on having an orgasm, there's just no manner of stimulation that's ever going to get them there—and there's definitely no way you're ever going to orgasm during the act of intercourse. The best gift you can give yourself is to make sure your head is in the right place. It's very simple: *I am looking forward to enjoying this delicious pleasure I am about to receive.* Here are some tips to get you where you need to be:

Get out of your head.

It's not time to balance your checkbook or worry about how the babysitter will be paid. Somehow the gutters will get cleaned, but if this is where your head is now, your mind is definitely in the wrong gutter. Think sexy thoughts. Fantasize. I know you know how.

Time it right.

I think it's safe to say that three minutes before the alarm clock goes off and the kids start tearing through the house as you begin the mad rush to get everyone where they need to be is not the right time to think about having an orgasm during intercourse.

Get rid of distractions.

No cell phone, regular phone, BlackBerry, laptop, TV (unless it's got a sexy visual going on) are permitted in your O zone. Get rid of these by at least putting them in the next room!

Learn to let go.

No one having sex with you at this very moment cares what kind of face you're going to make when you climax or any of the noise that may come out of you. In fact, the person having sex with you right this minute can't wait to see how all the more beautiful you become when you come. And the noises just amp up that excitement—for you and for your lover. Let your orgasm take you over and savor the feeling of handing over control to it.

For a Clitoral O . . .

Don't be afraid to use your own hands or fingers or a toy on yourself while your partner thrusts away at you. And if you'd like him to do any of the above, ask him. I'm sure he will oblige—and happily.

For a G-Spot O . . .

Take care to give this area foreplay before intercourse. Also, here's a neat trick that involves one of those "innocent" household sex toys we talked about: a pillow. In missionary, place a pillow under the lower half of her back, which tilts her pelvis forward. This is a great way for her to achieve a G-spot orgasm in this position. And note: He should not get too fixated on "aiming for her belly button" here. At this angle, every thrust will stimulate and massage the G-spot—and there's no way you can miss it using this technique.

Control the speed.

Go slow when you need to and fast when you want to. It's up to you what feels right.

Don't psych yourself out.

Quit saying "This isn't working. I can't have an orgasm like this!" and start saying things like "I wonder what could happen if I tilted my pelvis just a little to the left right here . . ."

YOU WANT MY LEGS *where?*

The rest of this chapter is all about sexual positions—the ones that can most increase the likelihood of orgasm and intensify the experience of orgasm for females! I highly recommend couples read through these together and talk them through together so they're both sure they really know what's going on. Missing out on a detail could mean missing out on an orgasm.

I know you have tried most of these positions before, but don't dismiss what's written here because you think you know it all already. Each of these positions listed here has been modified in one way or another to make them more orgasmic.

THE *missionaries*

Many people dismiss missionary as being "an old standby" or the position that requires the least imagination, but when it's performed with a woman's pleasure in mind, it can be one of the most orgasmic positions she can be placed in.

Standard missionary has the woman on her back with her lover facing her, on top, and between her spread, lifted legs. If he enters her at a higher angle, with his thrust coming from above her instead of just a basic in and out, he can actually rub his penis against her clitoris. If he starts low and thrusts upward, he can aim for the G-Spot. If he enters her in the missionary position on a perpendicular angle rather than at a more traditional quasi-parallel angle, he can massage her clit with his thumb while he is penetrating her—and even use a vibrating bullet on and around her clitoris during sexual intercourse. Trojan now also makes a new finger vibe called Vibrating Touch, which is perfect for this maneuver.

Here's another variation. Instead of opening her legs to accept him, she keeps them closed, meaning he's going to have to squeeze himself in, and that means excellent friction for all. To make the most of it, he should rub the tip of his penis against her clitoris for a while before he enters her—back and forth, side to side. Throughout, she will need to continue to keep her legs closed as tightly as she can manage as he thrusts inside of her. This is also a great technique for rear-entry positions—but we'll get into that in a bit.

In another missionary "legs together" variation, she lies on her back with her legs together and he enters slowly for ten long thrusts (long meaning counting to three going in and counting to three pulling out). Then, switch back to standard missionary, her legs wrapped around him, and he takes ten shorter thrusts. Switch back and forth several times until she explodes into orgasm.

Also starting in missionary, in this position she lies on her back, both legs together, but this time bent at the knee. She rests both legs over either his right or left shoulder as he enters her. Here's a tip: The shoulder chosen should be the *opposite* shoulder of the side of her clitoris that is most sensitive. For example, if the left side of her clitoris is more sensitive, she'll put her legs over his right shoulder and vice versa. Because she is getting more friction on one side or the other, she will get the stimulation she needs to climax that much faster.

Of course, part of the thrill of missionary for a woman is the sense of being "taken," so play right into the submission aspect and let the fantasies and the orgasms roll! Here, her legs can be up or down—it doesn't matter because what we're interested in here is what her arms are doing. And really, they're doing nothing at all but being held back by him. Once inside her, he grabs her hands and stretches her arms out so her body essentially forms a T shape. With her arms pinned down, she is unable to control anything that happens to her—she cannot push him away or pull him closer—and her pleasure literally rests in his hands.

This variation is amazingly stimulating, both for its deep penetration and the delightful friction it provides. Here, she lies with her tush at the edge of the bed, her legs straight up in the air. He then enters her and begins thrusting lightly. As he thrusts, he holds her ankles in his hands and begins scissoring her legs by crossing them and opening them, crossing and opening. The movement of her legs stimulates the vaginal walls, as well as the entrance to the vagina, and also creates varied pressure on the penis. Fun for all!

Here's a tricky and fun position that's great for G-Spot stimulation. She's flat on her back, knees bent and held together. She raises her butt slightly and he kneels under it, so that her butt rests on the front of his thighs. She opens her legs at the knees and places one foot over each of his shoulders. She can either support herself by keeping her hands on the bed or by placing pillows under her back. His hands remain free and can hold her waist, which is a very sexy, manly, take-charge way to control the thrusting.

Here's a maneuver that can be done in many positions but seems to work best in missionary because that's when he has the most balance and control. Once inside her, he aims his penis first to the left side of the vagina for three long strokes and then takes three more strokes to the right. Then three to the left and three to the right, and so on. The rhythm it creates is guaranteed to rock both partners' worlds.

And, men, if you really want to show her "who's in charge" (haha), try this the next time you and your lover are in the moment: Just as she begins to climax, quickly remove your penis—then, as quickly and suddenly as you slipped out, push yourself back in and keep thrusting till completion. For many women, the interruption builds the sexual tension and actually adds to the strength of the orgasm.

RIDE 'EM, *cowgirl*!

In her book *The Case of the Female Orgasm*, Dr. Elizabeth Lloyd says women are and much more likely to have an orgasm while on top. That makes so much sense for so many reasons when you think about it. When you're on top, you control everything—the angle of penetration, the speed of thrusting, pretty much you're in charge of the way the boat rocks. But what if you're not comfortable with all that power?

I once had a client whom I'll call Stella who, throughout her whole sexual existence, could not have an orgasm unless she was on top. Then something changed in her. "I have been married five years, and I never had a problem being on top. Even when I was pregnant with Emma (her baby daughter) I still loved the feeling of looking down at my husband as he watched my body and got all turned on by me. But since I had the baby, I just don't feel like me anymore."

"Do you still take the lead?" I asked her.

She shook her head. "Oh no. I don't like the way my body looks now, and I can't imagine what Stan would think of me, blobby hippo that I am, jumping up and down on him. I don't think I could take the look in his eyes if he didn't find me as attractive as he used to before the baby."

"Have you tried to be on top?"

"Absolutely not. He's tried to make me, but I just can't do it."

"Because he knows that's when you climax best."

"Sure. I mean, he doesn't actually say that to me. He jokes with me and tells me he knows I like to be in control and all that. But I just don't feel comfortable about it right now."

"You should tell him that," I recommended, and she did. I had a feeling he would be supportive and he was. He told her he thought she was absolutely beautiful, even more beautiful than when they first met, and that he loved her body just as it was. But he also understood that she had to feel right about it, so he made some suggestions. They tried it with the lights off, they tried it with him blindfolded, and when the stress of him seeing her was lifted, she was able to climax again.

"That's great," I told her. "But there's still a ways to go." We talked about self-esteem and body image and spent a good deal of time working on how to improve hers. It didn't happen overnight, but eventually she was able to take command again—and in full view.

WOMAN ON *top*

Here are some of the positions Stella and Stan and many of my other clients have tried. Sample each and see which ones might also work for you.

As I said, the woman-on-top position can be super orgasmic, but only if you control it in the way that feels best for you. You need to be comfortable and you need to be stable: There's nothing like losing your balance and toppling over in the heat of the moment only to lose the buildup!

As you straddle him, facing forward, rest your hands on either side of him and change the angle of entry by leaning forward, making sure his penis upon entry rubs up against your clitoris back and forth.

Now try straddling him facing his feet! Grab his ankles and slide yourself up and down. Or, instead of simply sliding up and down, make a figure eight motion with your hips.

Or try this: When you mount him as he's lying down, don't kneel around him, but squat. You can face him or swing around and ride him into the sunset. You probably want to work out your lunges and squats at the gym before trying this one to make sure your legs are nice and strong and ready to go the distance.

Bring some props into the mix—a stool or a chair can be great fun! He sits on the stool. Then you sit facing him with your legs wrapped around his waist. He places one hand on your back and the other on your tush. Before you begin grinding away, do those Kegels—at least twenty or thirty of them, however many of you can manage—as each of you savor the sensation. When it becomes too much to stand, by all means start having sex. Just keep squeezing while you do.

Now sit him down in a big roomy chair and sit yourself on top of him, facing him. Lean back and place your legs over his shoulders, letting them drape over the back of the chair. As he holds on tight to your hips as you grind, you'll both be getting a great workout—and not to mention the amazing G-spot stimulation for you.

And here's another great way to use the chair. He sits legs apart on the edge and you get on top of him, facing him, your legs wrapped tightly around him. He places his hands on your waist. Now, instead of the usual "in and out motion," you rotate and grind on top of him as he helps maneuver you. A great way to get the clitoral stimulation you crave!

BY *your* SIDE

Nothing's cozier than spooning. But did you know just how orgasmic these positions can be? Try lying down together, both of you on the same side of the bed and facing outward, with your back against his chest and so on. When he enters you, begin stimulating your clitoris with your fingers or hand—or can he do it for you. You could also use a vibrating bullet or pocket rocket as you rock back and forth. Whatever makes you happy!

Vary that initial position of you lying on your back with a small pillow tucked under your butt and your legs raised. He'll lie perpendicular to you, with one leg straight, one leg bent, and the bent leg hovering over one of your legs, creating an X. Hold your legs in their air as he thrusts; if you become tired, you can also bring your legs down. Vary this by keeping the same position but bending your legs at the knees over his pelvis. Then, swing both of your legs over his hips, giving his penis direct access.

I had another client, Jane, who finally just gave up trying to have having orgasms during sex. She was putting just too much emphasis on it and she realized she was taking the fun out of sex for her and her husband, Jeff.

Then guess what happened? She started having them. Her very first one was in this spooning position we just talked about. "I was really embarrassed to use toys with Jeff," she admitted. "But something just clicked this morning. We had just woken up and started to spoon, and that led right to sex. It was early in the morning and I was facing my night stand table and I just out of nowhere thought, 'What the hell. I'm going to reach into that drawer and grab my pocket rocket and go for it.' I don't think I'll ever give embarrassment so much as a second thought again!"

BACK IN *action*

Doggy-style is a daring position but also an intensely satisfying one for men and women both. For men, the penetration can't be beat. For women, the penetration is also a plus, especially if the penis is angled in such a way as it can hit the G-Spot. The depth of penetration this position allows also helps women achieve the cervical O. But as we talked about earlier, you have to be very gentle when you come in contact with the cer-

vix. If your lover gets overwhelmingly excited in this position, it might not be something you want to try on all fours.

The next time you make love in the doggie-style position (and we're talking rear-entry *vaginal* here, not anal), try this: As he thrusts inside, he should reach around and stimulate your clitoris with one hand, and with the other, he can lightly grab your butt cheek and push it out to the side. Now, with every thrust he makes, he pushes your tush to the side, which adds just a little bit of butt action to the mix and makes for some interesting sensations.

Even if you love doggie-style, it can sometimes be uncomfortable as we all well know. But that's no reason to rule it out. You just need to adjust it to meet your comfort level. Here are a couple of ways: In the first variation, she keeps her legs together with his on the outside of hers. In the second, she keeps her legs apart but rests her arms, head, and chest on a pillow and raises her tush up in the air. To really enhance the experience, he should not just "pound" away at her. He should gently stroke her shoulders and breasts and kiss her neck, face, and lips.

My client Amanda hated the doggie-style position, but it was Henry's favorite. She didn't want to have anything more to do with it, but his persistence drove them in to my office.

"Let's start by understanding what it is you hate about it," I told her.

She was quiet a moment before she responded. "Actually," she said, "I didn't always hate it. It used to be a great way for me to have an orgasm during sex. It's just recently that it's become a turn off."

"Was there something specific you can remember that may have turned you off from it?"

"No, not really. I think it may be because he always wants to do it that way, and I think I might need a little variety. Also . . . I find it a little demeaning," she said, and looked at Henry. "I'm sorry," she told him, and they both looked to me.

"Well, I definitely get the needing-more-variety part," I told them. "That's an easy one and I think you can pretty much work through that on your own." They both smiled and looked away. "But we should get to the heart of why you find it demeaning, Amanda," I said.

"Well, it's really just because when he's thrusting away like that . . . I don't know . . . it just seems so anonymous, you know? There's no intimacy or connection there. It's like he could be doing it with anyone."

"Ah, what do you think about that, Henry?"

"I dunno. I guess I do get pretty into it. I never felt like I wasn't being close to her though."

"It's like we have no connection as a couple when we do it that way," Amanda interrupted. "He gets all animalistic and cold with me. He never kisses me during doggie-style, and sometimes he hurts me."

"I hurt you?"

"I know it's not on purpose," she continued. "I think he just gets caught up in the moment and doesn't hear me when I yell 'Ouch!'"

"Have you ever talked about this before?"

"No," Henry said, and now he looked hurt.

"What if you were to try it again, Amanda, now that he knows what to do?"

"I guess," she said.

"And, Henry, do you think you could try and make it more romantic? Maybe kiss her or hold her, or even stimulate her if she wants you to?"

"Sure," he said. "Of course."

And that's what they did. I suggested they start off in other positions first and lead up to doggie-style. If she didn't want to do it just then, he wasn't permitted to press her about it and she wasn't arbitrarily supposed to refuse him. If they made it to the position, he was to keep the thrusting slow unless she asked for him to speed up, and he was to use his hands to stroke and caress her neck, shoulders, back, and tush.

I told him to kiss her a lot, on the lips, on her neck, down her back, and use words. "Tell her how wonderful she feels and how beautiful she is," I told him. "And call her by her name." The last part was key because it really served to connect them and prove to her that she is not just anybody when they are making love in that position. And happily, once the situation became more loving, Amanda craved the position more and more, and it went from anathema to nirvana. And speaking of nirvana . . .

kama sutra!

The *Kama Sutra* may be ancient, but its secrets are as yummy for lovers today as they were thousands of years ago. Here are a few of my favorite positions from the ancient text—the ones I feel that work best for women seeking to have orgasms during the act.

The Milk and Water Embrace

Here, the man lies on the edge of the bed, his legs hanging over the side, and the woman straddles him, facing him, her hands planted by his shoulders, her knees on each side of his pelvis, her feet alongside his legs. She can also kneel or squat over him—whatever way feels best.

Suspended Congress

In this challenging standing position, he stands with his back against a wall and she faces him, wrapping her arms around his neck, then jumps up to wrap her legs around his waist. She keeps her knees bent and rests her feet on the wall. She controls the action by rocking back and forth as she pushes her feet against the wall.

The Goat's Posture

A side-entry position, she lies on her side and stretches out her bottom leg. He crouches himself down between her thighs, kneels inside the bottom leg and lifts her top leg over his back. Now he enters and thrusts, all the while supporting her arms and shoulders. Here he can use his free hands to stimulate her as much as she desires.

AN *hour* IN HEAVEN

The conventional wisdom is that the average sex session lasts fifteen to twenty minutes. So how can you improve on that? You can start by devoting more time to it by spending less time making dinner or paying bills—or even on Facebook over the course of the day. Then when it comes to quality time with your lover, it isn't something you have to rush or squeeze in when you can. Admit it, watching TV together isn't spending quality time with your loved one. But we have to switch our priorities around. Time with your lover has to take precedence over a sink full of dirty dishes. Time with yourself, loving yourself, can surely be a priority over answering your e-mail. It's important to start changing the focus in your life, to re-view the way you see things. Because the more time you spend focusing on your orgasmic self, the more orgasmic you are going to be—even during intercourse.

In the next chapter, you'll be introduced to all kinds of ways to shift yourpriorities, but first there's a game you must try before you have any kind of sexual relations tonight.

Place a timer at your bedside and set it for fifteen minutes. All I want you to do for fifteen minutes is for each of you to get undressed.

Slowly. Languorously. Sexily. Watch your lover as he removes every article of clothing, piece by piece. Revel in the delight you give him as you remove each piece of clothing adorning you. Stand across from each other naked and really look at each other until the timer goes off.

Now set it again for another fifteen minutes, and this time I want you to lie together naked on the bed. Here's the big caveat: No Touching! You can fantasize and share your thoughts as you lie there naked together, but you are forbidden to be anywhere near each other.

When the timer runs out, set it again—and again for fifteen minutes. Now you are permitted to touch, but not in an overtly sexual way. You are allowed to kiss, you are allowed to gently stroke each other, and you can even hold each other if that's what you wish. You can tease around your partner's sexy parts with your fingers or your mouth, but you cannot touch these parts directly.

When the timer goes off again, prepare yourself for the final fifteen minutes. Now is your time to let go and be free. Stimulate her clitoris, touch his penis, lick, kiss, stroke, delight. As the timer runs down, see how long you can go without penetration. And once you have penetration, see how long you can hold out without any bumping or grinding or thrusting of any kind.

When the timer goes off again, you now have my blessing to go totally wild. But can you last another fifteen minutes before you just have to orgasm? I don't think you will!

BE IN THE *moment*

The last point I want to make in this chapter is a big one, so listen up. I taught an Orgasm 101 class for women a few years back, and when it came time for the Q & A, the thing those women wanted to know the most was if there was anything else they could do in any of the positions

I talked about to increase their chances of orgasms aside from what I'd already mentioned. Here it is: Whatever you do, don't just sit there or lie there. Be a part of what's going on with you. Make it happen for you. Rock your pelvis. Rotate your hips. Make circular motions with your pelvis, figure eights; whatever it takes, *I want you to take it.* I want you to try anything you can. Lift your hips up or in a circle. Grab your lover's hand or the back of his head. Whatever it takes, I want you to do it. And I want you to feel safe and comfortable and connected enough to know you can.

NOW *you* KNOW

For a woman, having an orgasm during intercourse is not as simple as snapping your fingers and making it so, but it's also not impossible. Whether you rely on strategic penile penetration or you break out some tools to help you along, these techniques can help you to experience the amazing feeling of orgasm coming over you. The electric bond you feel during orgasm, as your lower regions clench and release around your partner's member, is an experience worth all the careful practice. It's a feeling like no other.

To get there, again, connection and communication are key. Without them, having an orgasm during intercourse will be impossible. That's just the way it goes. In the next chapter, I will provide all kinds of ways for you to keep the fire and the closeness going in your relationship. Discover, learn, and above all else, enjoy!

CHAPTER 8

KEEPING THE *O* IN YOUR LIFE

"Everyone should live to be 92 years old, have an orgasm and drop dead. "
—JON CARROLL

Y ou know orgasms are good for you, physically, emotionally, psychologically, and you know why. You also know how to have an orgasm now, by yourself or with a partner, and using all manner of body parts and other implements. The last obstacle then is the "when."

How often should you have an orgasm? At least once a day, yes. Can you skip a day? Sure. But not too many days. What you want to do is make it a habit. Build having orgasms into your routine. You brush your teeth at least twice a day. You shower and you brush your hair and you moisturize. All that takes time, but you wouldn't even dream about leaving the house without doing these things.

If you can make time to jump on the treadmill or go to the gym, you can make time to have an orgasm. If you can squeak out twenty-five minutes to watch your favorite TV show, you can squeak out an orgasm (and in less time, the more you practice). The idea is to make it a priority. Place having orgasms closer to the top of your list (above vacuuming and washing the dinner dishes at the very least) and you will be a happier, healthier, sexier you.

In this chapter, we'll also find lots of creative ways to get your partner in on your "health plan." I'll even give you some worksheets to clock your progress. Once we're done with this chapter, you'll be an orgasm machine!

---

quick fix } TAKE THE PRESSURE OFF

When having an orgasm is not the be all and end all of the pleasuring you are giving yourself or receiving from your partner, you may actually clinch that O quicker and more powerfully.

CLEAR THE *emotional* DECKS

To live a fully satisfying, highly orgasmic life, you first have to clear space in your life to properly welcome the "new." This has to be done physically, meaning actually working sex and orgasms into your schedule, and also mentally. We'll get into the planning a bit later. For now, it's time to take a deep look into the closet of you and your psyche. To sweep away the debris and open up any "boxes" you've been storing away or hiding. Here's what to do.

Release yourself of any and all shame you may harbor about sex.

There's no worse buzz kill for a satisfying sex life than residual feelings of guilt or shame you might be carrying around from your past. These may have been taught to you by an adult who misguided you (sex is dirty!) or your religion (sex is a sin!). Or, you may have had an encounter or experience that instilled these feelings in you, perhaps a particularly awkward, early sexual encounter. It's amazing, but these kinds of experiences have a huge impact on who we become sexually as adults.

Were you pressured into having sex the first time? Were you unfavorably judged on your skills and abilities? Was there any enjoyment in it for you? Was the experience one you shared with others, or did you hide it deep within yourself? Or, in the most extreme situations, do you feel guilt or shame because of a situation of molestation or abuse?

Once you come to terms with the "what," you can take back control over your sexual situations. Can you pinpoint these issues on your own? Write them down on a sheet of paper that you can either burn or shred to tiny bits. Or are they not quite apparent and tangible for you—more like you have a sense of shame surrounding sexuality but you can't exactly say why you do?

Even for the lighter issues, it is probably a good idea to seek some level of therapy, to release yourself from these desire demons, and open your mind and your body to all the wonderful, healthy pleasures sex has in store for you. Painful memories of sexcapades past do not need to infect your enjoyment. Find what they are, speak to a friend or therapist, and banish them from your life and your bedroom once and for all.

Nancy was in her late thirties when she first came to see me. Since becoming sexually active around age thirteen, she had had a lot of sex and a lot of different partners. She was seeking my advice because she was married now, and while she said she was enjoying sex with him, she wasn't really able to have orgasms with him.

"After sex, I pretty much head to the bathroom, telling him I want to 'clean up a little.' I turn on the faucet so he can't hear me, and I give myself my own orgasm. I'm really not feeling that comfortable about it," she said, "but I'm also not comfortable talking to him about it. I really want to have an orgasm with him. I just don't know how."

I advised Nancy to take down her own sexual history—to write down every sexual experience she could ever remember having and how she'd felt after every experience, whether she'd felt euphoric or simply good or bored or uncomfortable or ashamed. Whatever the first emotion was that she associated with the experience that popped into her head, I advised her to go with that.

"That's a lot to remember," she laughed, but agreed to write down as much as she could recall and bring the list back with her for her next appointment.

We worked through Nancy's history, which took several sessions. We went through each experience and discussed them at length. At the end of our last session, we had determined that due to the volume of her escapades, she actually felt a bit of shame about her sexual past and didn't feel like she was worthy of pleasure with her husband who had a minimal sexual past.

A couple of months later, she wrote me an e-mail saying that this experience had been so healing for her that she was able to love and accept herself and finally enjoy her husband and herself sexually and orgasmically.

If you're "stuck" on what might be holding you back orgasmically, you may find doing this kind of exercise on your own helpful as well.

Relax, Rid, Rejuvenate

Another giant bedroom buzz killer: stress. Stress is insidious; it feeds on itself and only gets bigger and bigger if you let it. It has one mission: It wants to ruin your life. It wants to destroy you from the inside out. You can't let it. Because not only is it bad for your sex life, it's terrible for your overall health. You have to learn to let go of it.

I know, that's easy to say, less easy to control, but it is in your control. No, you can't always control the chaos that swarms you and tries to infect you with the stress, but you can control how you respond to it and take it in—or not. You have to work at it, but it will be worth it.

Can you name ten things you like to do to relax? Even five? How about one. Even in the most hectic of lives, there's at least one small space you can crawl into and escape the madness of your life for a while. If you only have one, great. Do it as often as possible. And while you are doing it, and you're mind is freeing up because it's not being tasked to worry about so many other things, see where else it leads you. For example, if you like meditation, try and imagine yourself doing yoga or painting or something else that can help ease the stress in your life. Take time for yourself each day to treat yourself to some relaxed time, and your mind and your body will be much more receptive to sex and orgasms than you ever imagined.

Love Yourself

Do you love yourself? Are you happy? If you find yourself to be depressed more often than not, it's time to sit back and evaluate why. You have to work on getting past whatever it is because the apathy and lack of enthusiasm for life that comes along with depression is creating a vicious cycle—inhibiting you from feeling sexy and getting the mojo you need to kickstart you right back on your happy path.

Do you find yourself to be desirable? Do you love and fully accept yourself? How you feel about yourself does affect your sexuality. It's important to do the work here to get you to the place of full and loving acceptance of yourself. It makes a big difference. Your thoughts are everything! There are some great self-esteem workbooks, workshops, and therapists so seek them if you need them.

SET THE *stage*

Now that you have your emotional space all cleaned up and organized, what about the physical? Part of feeling sexual means feeling "sexy." It doesn't mean you have to glob on the eye makeup and lipstick and teeter around in clear plastic stiletto stripper's heels (unless you want to, of course). It means feeling sexy in your own skin. And the best place to start is, again, from the inside out.

Take care of your body and it will reward you. Look after your health and you will reap so many benefits. Abuse yourself by gluing your tush to the couch, and you'll find that sex (and most activities for that matter) will hold little to no allure. Your goal is to provide yourself with the best possible physical environment possible for sexual enjoyment. And it's less much less complicated to do this than you may think.

Work Out Regularly

Orgasming is all about blood flow—and can you guess what else is? That's right: cardio. Experts recommend a good thirty minutes of cardio a day to keep all our systems flush and running. If you can't go to the gym, take a brisk walk. If you don't have a half hour to spare, find ways to keep active and moving. Park as far away from your office building as possible. Never use an elevator or escalator if you can help it: take the stairs. (Of course, if you work on the twenty-fourth floor this is probably not an option, but there are other ways.) Don't pick up the phone or send an e-mail to a coworker across the floor or on another floor. Physically pick yourself up out of your desk chair and walk, briskly, over to get the information you need.

Cardio is one element, flexibility and strength are the others, and each has an important role to play in sexual performance and your enjoyment of it.

Consider how important flexibility is in getting "just the right friction" going with your partner. The more you are able to bend and stretch, the more luck you're going to have hitting the sweet spot. You're also going to be a lot more comfortable while you're at it—and less likely to injure yourself at that. Consider a pretzel as an example. You can shape malleable dough into any shape you want, but once it's hardened, if you try and move a section of it into a different angle, that part's just going to snap and break!

Yoga and Pilates are wonderful ways to experience the trifecta of exercise—and yoga is also something of a natural aphrodisiac. Did you know that? It's true. It calms your mind, relaxes the soul, and lightens the spirit. And when you perform some of your more provocative postures for your partner in the nude, well, the sky's the limit on arousal—for both

of you. If you have a full-length mirror nearby, even better. Ask your partner to join you, explaining that yoga has been proven to increase blood
flow to all areas of the body —and is supposed to ignite the libido. Invite
your partner to test it out with you and see if you can prove the ancient
wisdom—over and over again.

As far as strength goes, remember some of the amazing positions
we covered in the last chapter? You're not going to be able to do some of
the more challenging ones if you're not strong enough to support your
own weight! Here's an exercise I created for my last book, *A Little Bit
Kinky*, that can actually help you build strength and get more sexually
fit.

Love Muscles

It's no secret that fit people have more fabulous sex. But did you know
there are specific muscles you can exercise that will directly affect your
performance and experience in the bedroom? It's true. Your butt and
lower abdomen elevate the pelvis and make it easier for you to have close
contact with your lover, and inner thigh muscles can actually compen-
sate for weak vaginal muscles. When in the act, contracting the thighs
and butt together can squeeze the penis, giving both partners added
pleasure. And strong pelvic floor muscles make for more intense orgasms—and who doesn't want those?

Here are three excellent exercises that you can do to strengthen
those love muscles. For maximum effect, do at least fifty of each every
day.

1. Lie on your back, knees bent, hands behind head, and lift your upper
   body by crunching up your abdomen.

2. Lie on your back, knees bent, shoulders on floor, and raise just your pelvis off the floor. Hold and squeeze for a count of thirty—or as long as you can hold at first, and work up to thirty—and more.

3. Lie on your back with your legs straight up in the air and held together. Now slowly let them drop to the sides, spreading them as far apart as you can, and slowly pull them back together.

Check Yourself Out!

Actually, that's important and we'll talk more about that in just a bit, but what I mean here is to *get yourself checked out* by a doctor at least once a year. (And definitely not less than twice a year by your gynecologist if you're on the pill or have an IUD.)

Familiarize yourself with health issues common for women in your age group, and don't be afraid to ask questions from your doctor if you have any—that's what she's there for. If there is a pressing health issue, letting it hang over you is only going to cause you stress (remember that ugly pest!), which is going to block the mental part of you that experiences sex. Not to mention what ignoring a health problem can do to the physical side of things. When you're grappling with unexplained pain or exhaustion, who wants to think about sex? You take your car in for servicing when the sticker says it's time. Why not you?

Eat Real Food

There can be a beautiful marriage between food and sex, and we'll actually get into some sexy foods and arousing food play in just a bit. But there's another side to the coin—where the foods you eat can negatively impact your performance and your pleasure when it comes to sex.

VITAMIN O

Do you pay attention to what goes into your mouth on a daily basis? Are you a takeout queen or processed food princess? Are you addicted to sugar? Really paying attention to what you eat is going to make you better sexually for one very important reason: energy. I know you know this. Bad food fills you up but weighs you down. Good food gives you consistent energy, so by the end of even a long day, you might yet be up for a raucous romp—and not in a coma from a sugar crash.

Investigate foods and their nutritional value. Pay attention to calories—earned and burned. The higher quality of stuff you take in, the higher quality you're doing to draw out.

I had a client who was a petite five foot three but nearly two hundred pounds. When Ali came to see me in her late thirties, she was a virgin. "I've never really considered myself to be a sexual person, and I've never really dated," she told me. "It's not like I haven't wanted to or anything, it just never happened for me."

It was important for me to be as direct and honest with her as possible, and we began a discussion about her weight. Aside from the obvious health risks she was putting herself in, we talked about the other-risks she was in danger of because she had shut herself off sexually. "I couldn't imagine being with someone else in that way at my size. I'm not even interested in myself like this," she said.

When you're ready , sometimes a push is all you need, and Ali decided that day to enroll in a weight loss program. Within six months, after eating well and exercising, her weight started to melt away.

As soon as she got to a comfortable weight, she started to feel sexual. But with little experience, she was also a little scared. We met several times over the course of a year, and in that time we covered all the essentials, from how to date to how her body worked, sexually speaking.

Ali began experimenting with masturbation and became hooked. "It feels so good," she told me, "but not just at the time. I find if I give myself an orgasm before getting out of bed in the morning, I don't need to bother with coffee!"

Once she was feeling sexually confident, she felt ready to date. Three years later, she's happily married, enjoying a deeply satisfying sexual relationship, and she's also working as a part-time Pilates instructor. Better health through orgasms!

GET *into* YOURSELF

When it comes to having orgasms, there is only one person that truly matters, and that person is you. Above, we talked about how feeling good about yourself leads to better sex and better orgasms. Here are some ways to show yourself how much you matter sexually, and keep your brain focused on yourself as a sexual being that deserves all the pleasure in the world.

Buy Yourself Some Sexy Things

There is nothing sexy about your old threadbare underwear. Even if you're single and you rationalize "No one's going to see this," just know that *you* see it. All day long, you walk around with a subconscious image of yourself as a person who's not worthy of pretty underthings—and who is not desirable enough that anyone else would want to see them. Very bad.

The same goes for overwearing underwear like granny panties, Spanx, or other practical but unflattering bloomers. True, we all need smoothing with our Spanx in some outfits—but they are meant for form-fitting dresses and that kind of thing. Not to wear under your jeans like armored boxer shorts. A lace thong may ride up from time to time, but at least it reminds you that it's there, and slipping into places so many other wonderful things could be. Haven't you ever been rubbed the right way by a pair of panties? That just can't happen when they droop!

(Researchers in one sex study discovered that wearing (and actually walking around in) two-inch heels daily can help improve the strength of a woman's pelvic muscles.)

Pleasure Yourself

Yes, this is so important that I spent an entire chapter on it, but it begs repeating—again and again and again. The only way you're ever going to be able to show someone else how to "play" you like the beautiful pleasure instrument you are is to know how you work—what does it for you and what doesn't. And the only way for you to know this with certainty is experimentation and plenty of practice.

I asked some of my clients what gets them going. Do any of these methods they talk about below work for you? Try them out—each and every one!

"I like to use a pillow or two and lie on top of them and thrust into the pillow with my hand stimulating my clit at the same time and if this doesn't work I add a vibrator and place it on the pillow and rub up on it."

—Alice, thirty-six

"When I pleasure myself, I always keep legs apart and I usually leave my underwear on. I start rubbing my clitoris light and slow, then harder and harder, faster and faster. I can feel my wetness coming through my underwear and that's when I know an orgasm is on its way."
—Roxanna, twenty-eight

"I start by stimulating my clitoris with one hand, and then I place one or two fingers inside of me and start stroking myself back and forth. Sometimes I'll pull them out and stimulate my clit again. But sometimes I'll use both hands, one stimulating my clit while I slide the fingers of the other in and out of my vagina. Sometimes I'll take either hand away from what it's doing and use it to massage my breasts and nipples. I also like to do this in front of the mirror—but I only like to look at my body not my face."
—Judy, forty-six

"When I'm taking a bath is when I usually masturbate. I like to place my legs under the running water for foreplay and then I finish myself off with my fingers on my clitoris rubbing them quickly back and forth in a sideways motion until I come."
—Annie, thirty-three

"If I want to come quick I use a vibrating bullet on my clit and imagine some random man going down on me."
—Linda, fifty-three

Just remember: Practice, practice, practice. Getting yourself off is the one activity you can do over and over again and never get sick of.

Know Your Body

I want you to introduce yourself to each and every inch of you; then I want you to fall in love with yourself. We covered some of this in the self-pleasuring chapter. I want you to know what your ankles feel like and if they're at all sensitive. I want to explore how deep your belly button is, and whether or not it tickles to be touched on the other side of your knees. I want you to investigate how much pressure you can apply to pinching your nipples before it goes from delightfully sensitive to *Ouch!* I want you to know what your vagina feels like—the canal. I want you to examine the shape and the texture. I want you to stimulate yourself with your own fingers while you hold a finger inside yourself and experience for yourself the amazing contractions that make up an orgasm. (Trust me, after this, you will never fake it again.) And while you're at it, be sure to keep up those Kegels!

Keep an Open Mind

There are many ways to orgasm. If you're not finding just the right way with your hands, there's absolutely nothing wrong with playing with a sex toy to get you to where you want to be—and that goes for being by yourself or with a partner. The key here is *whatever works*. If you like a Realistic dildo, go for it. A vibrating bullet. A Rabbit vibrator. Nipple clamps. A large cucumber—whatever works. You might want to keep an assortment of toys in a box under your bed (okay, just not the cucumber or anything else that's perishable) so you have quick access when the mood strikes.

howdy, PARTNER!

The key to having lots of orgasms in your life is to make it an integral part of your life. And if you're married or involved in a long-term relationship, you really have to make it the cornerstone of that relationship—the piece that holds it all together.

Couples get into ruts all the time. They use the ten minutes or hour they may have after the kids are asleep to talk about bills or grocery shopping or what Aunt Edna wants for Thanksgiving dinner. None of this is important—not first and foremost.

The next time you and your partner have ten "alone" minutes together, forget about doling out chores that need to be done and exchange sexual fantasies instead. Or, just jump right in and enjoy each other. Make connecting physically the first thing on your list. Once you're all sweaty and hot and out of breath, then decide who's going to take little Janie to the birthday party at the climbing gym on Saturday afternoon. Because if you get to that stuff first, you're just going to squash any desire to get to the good part!

Sex is not something you do because you've run out of minutiae to itemize. Time to change your focus! And once you make the shift and give it this kind of amazing prominence, once you make your sex life feel loved and respected and cherished, it will reward you again and again.

Another way to amplify the importance of sex in your relationship is to make a bet about something—a sporting event, the weather, what one of your kids will say next—with the winner being granted a mutually agreed-upon sexual favor. It could be one hour of being a sex slave, a full-body massage, or even an oral favor. It's entirely up to you.

TEASE FOR *two*

Teasing makes the heart—and the titillation—grow fonder and is arousing on both sides of the tease. The one who teases has control. Slip a provocative note in your lover's briefcase and you get him wanting you all day. Go one step further and "sext" (sex-text) him, complete with a naughty photo for you, and get your own self worked up thinking all day of how he's "suffering" at work when all he really wants to do is come home and jump on top of you—and how he's going to "punish" you for all that suffering you inflicted!

And you can enjoy a tease being done to you as much as you can when you inflict it on another. Encourage your lover to share his sexual thoughts and dreams with you—especially when there's no way possible you're going to be able to act on the luscious filth he's whispering to you while you're folding laundry with the kids watching cartoons in the same room.

The buildup to sex can be as fun and intense as the having of sex. So while you can't have sex right at these moments when you're teasing each other with the promise of it, the thinking about it is what's important—showing interest, being creative, having fun, and most importantly, connecting.

A *venture* TO ADVENTURE

Of course, you can have a wonderful sexual adventure with your partner right in your bed. But you can also venture outside, being creative and busting out of the bedroom from time to time.

You don't have to out and out do it in public, but you can certainly make salacious suggestions without ever saying a word.

One of my favorite ideas came from a friend of mine; I'll call her Audrey. It was her husband Joel's birthday, and while she had gotten him a couple of nice gifts, she really never felt like either of them was really "the gift"—the special one he'd remember year after year. Then she got a brilliant idea.

"I told him we were going out to dinner on me," she said, "and that I was going to take care of everything. Joel's kind of traditional and doesn't feel completely comfortable with the idea of a woman paying for his meal, but somehow he decided to go along with it. Anyway, after we had ordered dessert, I got up from the table.

"He lightly clutched my wrist. 'Where are you going?'

"I looked at him slyly and said, 'I'm going to find the waiter to pay the check before you intercept it from me.'

"He smiled. 'What makes you think I haven't paid it already?'

"'Because I told them to ignore you at all costs,' I said, smirking back at him.

"So I dropped off my credit card with the waiter (because I knew Joel would try and pay anyway) and I went into the bathroom. I slipped into one of the stalls. From my purse, I took out a neatly wrapped box and I opened it. I then slid out of my very tiny panties, slipped them into the box, and placed the box back in my purse. I headed back to Joel.

"When I arrived at the table, he was signing a credit card receipt. 'What happened here?'

"He smiled at me. 'The waiter came by and dropped it off while you were in the bathroom apparently,' he said. 'What took you so long?' he asked.

"I pulled the package out of my purse. 'Happy Birthday,' I said, and I tossed it at him.

"He opened the package just as the waiter had come to pick up the check. Both men went bright red, but mine smiled back at me as the waiter jumped to the next table. I knew from the look in his eyes that it was the high point of his day—and what went on when we finally got home proved it with a miraculous night of passion!"

While Audrey and Joel didn't actually do anything in public, having the hint of speculation that something could occur—that something crazy-sexy between them had gone public somehow—was hugely exciting for them both.

Have you ever had sex in a public place? I don't mean in the privacy of your car—as thin as that privacy is. I mean right out in the open for the world to see, but disguised enough so you keep 'em guessing.

Well, you don't really ever have to have sex in a public place to get that kind of charge. You don't even have to leave your house or your bedroom. I'm just encouraging you to shake things up a little. Have sex somewhere you've never had it before.

Surely you've tested out your living room couch. But how about the desk in your home office, or even your dining room table? Your laundry room? Your garage?

There's a whole world of erotic possibilities out there waiting for you when setting a scene for sensuality, and any room will do. Just keep it sexy!

Give Your Bedroom a Makeover.

Take a look around the space. Does it really present itself as a pleasure den? Or is more like a satellite home office, strewn with bills and paperwork, or a spare playroom laden with toys? Keep clutter to a minimum—especially passion killers like bills and school permission slips! Decorate in soft tones. Add votive candles in pretty holders. Keep artwork sexy. Photos of your kids are great to have, but these are not exactly going to put you in the mood—unless you're looking to make more of them.

Deck Out Your Closet.

Why not use your closet romantically if you have the space to spare. Drape silky scarves across the floor and bring in soft, incandescent lighting. Maybe in your closet, out of the reach of your kids, you can store an antique-looking trunk where you can keep toys and lubricants, lotions and oils, scarves and restraints, whatever you're into.

Looking-Glass Love Land.

And of course you don't have to go anywhere, not even out of your bedroom, to be transported to your own world. If you don't already have a large mirror in your bedroom, this would be a great place to install one! Place a soft blanket down in front of it, and remove all, or if you prefer, most of your clothes. How you proceed now and what you do together exactly is up to you. Just follow one rule: Keep eye contact with your partner's reflection. Now you have a secret lover in a faraway land who, when you think about it, is making you feel fantastic without even touching you from his side of the glass.

FOOD *fetish*

Food can be very sexy, and people have been experimenting with it in sexplay since the dawn of time. Some foods are considered sexy for their shapes (hello, Mr. Cucumber!), and with others, it's more about texture. Some are sexy because of the way you eat them (and feed them)—with your fingers. And some contain natural chemicals that are known to promote arousal. Whatever the reasons they work, aphrodisiacs are good, yummy fun. Here's a list of some of the top ones:

- lobster
- raw oysters
- sushi
- caviar
- artichokes
- avocados
- bananas
- cucumbers
- watermelon

- almonds
- chocolate
- ginger
- olive oil
- honey
- wine
- figs
- mangoes
- peaches

- strawberries
- celery
- cherries
- raspberries
- black currants
- pineapple juice

For your next date night, why not make a special bedroom picnic using only foods that can be served and savored using only your fingers. That doesn't mean you need to be confined to traditional finger foods, though. Be crazy. Be uninhibited. Don't be afraid to make a gorgeously gooey mess. So what? Think of all the fun you can have lapping it up—or having it lapped up—from all the naughty places it can spill or crumble or drip.

My friend Stacy recently did this with her husband, Ed. Before he left for work in the morning, she slipped a card into his briefcase to join her for a "Bare and Bawdy Bedroom Buffet" later that evening. For the rest of the day, she shopped for pretty candles and water-resistant covering for the bed. She decked out the space with pretty scarves and candles, dimmed the light, and made the centerpiece of the room the middle of the bed, where she laid out a frisky feast.

She and Ed spent the evening snacking and licking and kissing and nibbling. "I must have had six orgasms!" she told me over drinks several nights later.

candy-licious!

There's lots of sweet possibilities to embrace when candy's in the mix. Here are two of my favorites:

The Painter. Have your lover dip a paintbrush (or a collection of paintbrushes if you're into it) into a bowl of chocolate syrup. Then, guiding him with your words and soft moans, have him "paint" you with long, luscious strokes. He can paint all your sexy parts, and you teach him some of the ones that are less obvious. When he covers a part of you, have him lick you clean!

Sweet Spot. This one's also designed to teach your lover all about the places on you that crave his attention. Pour some M&Ms into a bowl on your night table. Lie down on the bed in front of your lover, reach your hand into the bowl, and scoop a few out. Place them wherever you please—your belly button, your nipples, your cleavage, even some on the area just above your pubes, your wrists, the inside of your elbow. Tell him to eat his dessert off of you—and to be sure he licks the "plate" clean!

ACTING *out*

Role play and fantasy are two great ways to get closer to your partner. For one, they involve a certain degree of trust. Opening up about a sexual fantasy with someone can be terrifying. And with role play, you really have to be comfortable with another person to pretend to be someone else and, most of the time, an exaggerated characterization of someone else in a sexual way with that person.

It forces you to open up to expressing yourself in new and exciting physical ways. It also challenges you to be vulnerable and, therefore, trusting with your partner. You're both in on the game and there are no judgments made—even in the most hilariously awkward moments. It isn't just about donning a costume and pretending to be someone else for a new sexual thrill. It's about pure fantasy and all that entails. And because each of these demands open communication and connection, they have been known to produce orgasms fairly quickly for those who chose to partake in them.

The hottest sexual situations are the ones that push you just outside the parameters of what you perceive is your comfort level. Think of it like exercise. You can feel good going at a steady, comfortable clip. But it isn't until you push yourself beyond where you think your limit is that you really hit the zone. Here are a few role play suggestions. The best ones will come right from you and your partner:

Sexy Strangers.

Arrange to meet your partner separately at a bar—or even a park, a bookstore, the zoo. It doesn't really matter where. When you get together, pretend you don't know each other. How this night will end is entirely up to you!

Naughty Nurse.

There are few outfits more fetishy than an old-fashioned nurse's uniform—even without sexing it up with an ultra-micro-mini uniform, thigh-high white lace fishnets, and platform heels. Of course, these "extras" are recommended. If you are the nurse, the power you'll feel wearing this outfit as you watch your patient writhe with desire under your doting care will be irresistible. And if you are the patient and your partner the nurse be sure to get all the carnal care you crave for your "cure."

Sexy Spy.

You are a top operative on a very important, highly dangerous mission. Mr. X is harboring top-secret information about a dastardly plot that could put the world in incomparable jeopardy. You are to use your special skills to seduce those secrets out of Mr. X and make him so hot with desire, that not only will he tell you everything, he'll switch sides to remain in service to you!

Saucy Schoolgirl.

You can't think of anything more boring than Mr. Q.'s chemistry class. You're dying to conduct your own chemistry experiment—and this one involves none other than sexy Mr. Q. himself. He's very strict; you know the only way to really get his attention is to sass him and infuriate him with your insolence. When class lets out and he tells you must stay after, he'll be sure to teach you the lesson you wanted to learn all along.

Stern Teacher.

From the other end of the classroom, you have a student who just won't cooperate. A class clown and a thug, he makes you crazy during your lectures—and for more reasons than he interrupts you constantly. He's a strapping young lad, and what he's really doing is calling out for you to set him straight—and if that means using a strap to teach him who's boss, well, that's entirely up to you.

Slutty Cheerleader.

The football team lost again, and you're the only one who can cheer the guys up. You have powers the other cheerleaders don't have—and you know how to use your mouth for more than cheers. Whether it's just the quarterback who needs a boost or the whole team—one by one, two by two (it's your fantasy after all!)—get in there and show your team spirit! (And if the football team won, just switch it around and make it the preparty celebration in the locker room!)

Ditzy Secretary.

Mr. Z is going to be so mad at you if he finds out you lost the F file again. He's told you time and again that you are the worst secretary he's ever had, and every time you mess up, your punishment gets more and more severe. Except, like Maggie Gylennhal in *The Secretary*, you have to admit you like Mr. Z's punishments and you probably mess up on purpose more often than not.

Bitchy Boss.

Can you believe that punk Johnny Rotten stole your account again? Made himself look good at your account in front of the board again! You don't have to take that from him. It's time to call him into your office, close the door (and lock it), and give him an on-the-job training session he'll never forget.

Merry Maid.

There's nothing you love more than scrubbing and dusting (this is a fantasy world, remember) and you're so proud of your recent polishing of the sideboard, you just have to call the boss in to admire your work. Now, he's either a clean freak like you, so he's so dazzled by your dusting he can't help but sweep you up in his arms and thank you in the most romantic way. Or he's a cruel sadist who can only see the fingerprint he left when he touched the banister and will now be cleaning up your act in his own deliciously deviant way.

Lusty Librarian.

Some people love books but you really love books. In fact, you love books so much you fantasize about making love on a pile of open books. The library's closed and won't be open for another half hour—why not indulge your fantasy, even if it's just you and your books. Spread them open, spread them out, then spread yourself and go to town! (Just remember that the janitor's shift hasn't ended yet, and he might be lurking between the shelves and watching.)

Horny Hairdresser.

There isn't a better head of hair you've ever worked on than Mr. L's luscious locks. Long and silky, "wasted on a man," you look forward to his appointments more than Christmas morning when you were a kid. Usually you can control yourself, but this time his hair is just irresistible. You just can't help yourself as you stroke the silken strands, lifting just a few and stroking them across your cheeks. He watches on in the mirror, clearly amused and into your delight. So you take it further. You begin to graze your neck and your shoulders. Your cleavage. Soon you are out of control, your clothes in a ball on the floor, and you are wrapped only in his hair, like Lady Godiva—but sexier in all the imaginative ways you're tarting it up with his tresses.

Misguided Masseuse.

You didn't pay very good attention at masseuse school, so when you start your new job at the Sensual Springs Spa, you figure you're just going to have to wing it. Lucky for you, your first client seems like a really nice guy, and he's sexy as hell. You oil up your hands with Sensual Springs Special Oils, and you get ready to run your hands all over the rugged textures of his tempting terrain. Except he's almost too tempting—the feel of his skin under your hands is starting to get you more excited than you ever imagined possible. As you run your hands over his shoulders and down the small of his back, he quickly turns over, and you can see he's sharing your excitement. And without those pesky guidelines getting in your way, you can earn your tip any way you like.

Sizzling Stripper.

You are an erotic dancer and you love what you do. You love the power you have over men, watching them watch you as you bend and twist, gyrate and dance. You love the anticipation as much as they do—especially when it comes to your favorite client. This hunky piece of man flesh dotes on you like you're the only one in the room every time he comes in. In fact, you can't remember him ever having had a lap dance from any of your girlfriends. And he's such a good tipper. You decide tonight's the night you're going to set him on fire with your performance, and you'll even toss those "no touching" rules right out the window for one night of forbidden passion and see where it leads!

Red-Hot Hooker.

You're the number one girl on the street, and it's no wonder why. No one wears spandex and sequins and thigh-high boots as well as you. That's why you make the big bucks, and why your clients, especially your return clients, never balk at your rates. You know how to show these guys the time of their lives, and your favorite ones are the really rich ones. Have you ever had your lover toss money at you while you're hot and heavily involved in pleasuring him or yourself? Try it out tonight!

pushing BOUNDARIES

There are levels past fantasy and role play just waiting for you to discover them. How much can you handle?

Maybe you have a fantasy about being in a threesome with your partner, but you don't really have the desire to bring another real live person into your bed. Here's a solution: Dial up one of those raunchy 900 numbers while you and your partner are going at it and see if another voice in the room, grunting and moaning, shrieking and screaming, will do the trick. Having a dirty movie on in the background is also another way to simulate this—but we'll get into that a bit later.

What about bondage? Have you ever fantasized about being captured and bound and taken over and over again "against your will"? Traditionally, S/M is a power play of dominant over submissive, of a "sadist" controlling the actions, but much to the "masochist's" delight. And that's the most important thing to remember. When you experiment with bondage, both partners, in whatever role, must ultimately feel *delight*. If there's anything else going on—coercion, fear, dread, anxiety—it's time to call it a day.

"My husband wants to experiment with bondage," Alexis, a fortyish mother of three, shared with me. "But I'm a little nervous about it. I mean, it's not that I'm not intrigued and excited about it. Even thinking about it makes me kind of tingly. But he's six foot five—and so much bigger and stronger than me. I'm worried that in the heat of the moment, I might end up getting hurt or something."

I assured her that her fears were valid, but that as long as she and her husband communicated properly, she would most probably be okay. "Decide on a safe word," I told her.

"A what?"

"A safe word is a word you both need to understand, something that stops the action. Saying things like 'no' and 'stop' and 'you're hurting me' fuel the fantasy. You need a word to take you out of the moment."

"Like what?" she asked.

"Well, I have some friends who use 'pineapple.'"

"Pineapple? My goodness. It doesn't get sillier than that!"

"Exactly!" I told her. Silly as anything, but that's what it takes.

If you push these boundaries together, whether you're the top or bottom, be aware of how your actions are affecting your partner. I strongly recommend that you don't drink heavily or take drugs for bondage play; it's extremely important to keep all your senses sharp, which will make the experience that much more pleasurable. Especially if you're thinking of filming it.

> Think porn is a guy thing?
> Think again! A recent study
> found that women get physically
> aroused by a much wider variety
> of erotic imagery than men do.

hey, WATCH IT!

Sex on screen freaks some people out, but if you're open to it, many women have reported having incredibly explosive orgasms while watching it. Porn is for foreplay. It's an "igniter" and a resource for ideas and new things to try. It can even help you out when you might not be totally "in the mood" and want to get there quickly.

Not all porn is equal. Some of it is definitely not made for us. Close-ups of body parts inserted in other body parts and messy "money shots" are made with men in mind (they are different creatures than us in many ways, after all). Porn that's too "hardcore" has even been known to have the opposite effect on women—turning them off for days or even indefinitely. But like I said, there are options that may be worth investigating.

Instructional "how to" videos are not technically considered to be porn, but they have been known to get many women revved up and ready to roll as they depict very real things going on to teach you how to repeat them.

"Softcore" porn is what generally appeals to women most. These are the adult movies that may have a more complicated story line than "the pizza man delivered—and *delivered*." They feature women with men, women with women, and sometimes there's a group effort going on, but there's nothing shocking or overtly graphic about the action.

And not all porn is movies. Magazines and the Internet are loaded with lusty visuals for you to flip to or click on. Here are some good adult websites:

- masturbationpage.com
- the-clitoris.com
- the-penis.com
- hustler.com
- playboy.com
- hotpornforwomen.com
- thecouplespleasuredome.com
- Sssh.com

For movies, look for a book called *The Ultimate Guide to Adult Videos* which can let you know quickly which movies you might want to check out—and which to fear with your very life! Here are a few that were made, for the most part, by women for women:

- Jenna Jameson's *The Masseuse*
- *Dinner Party,* directed by Cameron Grant
- *Five Hot Stories For Her by Lust Films*
- *Let's Get Physical by Playgirl*
- *101 Positions for Lovers by Jamye Waxman*
- *Pleasure Touch 1: Toying with Pleasure by Jamye Waxman*

JUST SHOOT *me*!

Sometimes it's fun to watch, and sometimes it's fun to dive right in! Take innocently naughty (that's "naughty in the eye of the beholder") photos of your lover and have him return the favor. Maybe he can photograph you lapping up an ice cream cone, or you can shoot him licking the pit in a peach. This all makes for excellent fun, subtle foreplay that your imagination makes hot.

Carrie was super shy and a bit introverted. She came to see me because she craved more attention from her husband—and not just sexual attention. She wanted to be taught how to play flirtatiously with him. One of my suggestions was to pull out a camera and have him take photographs of her. Her job was to make the photographs sexy and interesting.

"I had him take pictures of me dressing and getting undressed, eating, swimming, and sleeping," she said. "When I was eating, I'd make sure the meal I was eating was really sexy, like cherries I sucked the 'meat' off. Other fruits, like watermelon, I'd slurp up and let the juice drip out of my mouth and over my chin. Swimming, I'd jump out of the water and flash my breasts. I'd sunbathe naked and let him take any pictures he wanted to take. Sleeping, I'd wear my most erotic lingerie to bed, and when I was a little conscious, I'd position my body into very erotic poses. We had a great time!"

She and her husband, thanks to their camera and their creativity, found that they could take the most mundane everyday acts and make them erotic, playful, and flirty. They made a private album of their photo sessions, and it ended up being fun for both of them. She got the attention she wanted and turned this exercise into foreplay.

What about you? Can you take it up a notch? Will you play male photographer and lingerie model? Female photographer and wild man found in the jungle? Or just play it straight, each of you taking sexy photos of each other in various stages of undress? Whatever you decide, just enjoy yourself and be free about it.

MAKE A *game* OF IT

One of the least intimidating and most exciting ways to bring adult films into your relationship is to make a game of it—really capitalize on sharing the experience together. Here are some ideas:

Every time someone in the movie sighs "Oh God," beat your partner to the punch—with a light punch on the arm. Whoever throws the first punch earns one sexy kiss wherever they want, right then and there. Tally up the punches at the end of the film, and whoever's thrown the most gets to enjoy a long, luscious sexual favor at the expense of the loser. But truly, are there any losers here?

As you watch an adult movie together, list some notes, focusing on some of your favorite parts. When the movie ends, exchange your lists, see if there are any activities you can agree to try together, and get down to it.

During the movie, press Pause every time you see something you like and talk about why. Either show your partner why right there and then or prolong the ecstasy until after the movie—whatever the situation calls for.

Tie your lover to a chair and "force" him or her to watch *their* favorite porn scene—as you do your best to simulate it in the flesh.

What if regular movies or TV actually let you see what happened to characters when everything fades to black during a love scene? Why not make it up yourselves?

Speaking of games, here are some favorites of mine.

pleasure HUNT

This game, which you play naked, teaches you a ton about each other's bodies. To play, begin touching your lover everywhere—earlobes, nipples, toes, wherever—and have him or her rate how being touched in these places feels on a scale from 1 to 10. Pay careful attention and repeat touching as necessary. Then it's your partner's turn to explore. The point here is to take an inventory on each other's hot spots, at least once a month as they are subject to change. Do this and you'll always know just where to touch to keep the passion fresh.

peaking IT!

This is a masturbation game whose goal is not only to bring you to orgasm, but to make the one you end up having insanely intense. To start, either pleasure yourself or your partner needs to begin pleasuring you. As you feel yourself getting closer to climax, stop the action, take a deep breath, and pant to the count of ten. Now switch the kind of stimulation you were doing. If it was clitoral before, start stimulating G-Spot or nipples or anus. Again, as you become more and more excited, *stop*. Do the breathing exercise again. Now switch positions and try a new kind of stimulation. When you get close to climax, stop again, do the breathing, and so on—until you just can't take it anymore. Pretty much after five rounds of this, you are probably going to explode!

love STRADDLE

Strip down so you're wearing only your underwear. Now, you and your partner need to sit facing each other, holding hands, and straddling your legs as far apart as you possibly can without making yourselves uncomfortable.

He leans forward and you lean back for the count of five. Then you lean forward and he leans back for the count of five.

Make sure you can both feel your inner thigh and groin muscles stretching, but be careful: *It's not supposed to hurt*. Do this ten times before sex.

TEASE AND *please*

In the morning, stimulate yourself close to orgasm but don't allow yourself to have one. In the middle of the afternoon do the same thing. Then at night, go all the way with yourself or with your partner and see what a buildup can do!

hot AND COLD

Have an ice pack and a heating pad nearby. With your underwear on, place the ice pack over your vulva for eight seconds or for as long as you can stand it. Then do the same with the heating pad. Do this ten times with both the ice pack and the heating before sex or masturbation—and get your partner get involved!

yogasm!

We already talked about how sexy yoga can be and on so many levels. Physically, the poses put you in many delightfully carnal compromising positions. But there's also a physiological element. For example, poses like *upavista konasana*, a wide-legged straddle pose, increases blood flow to your Yoga and also helps strengthen your pelvic floor muscles—excellent for orgasms as we well know by now.

Here's how to do *baddha konasana* (which you should try to do five times before masturbation or sex):

Sit with your knees bent and the soles of the feet touching.

Lightly hold your big toes and lean your torso forward over your legs, keeping your back gently rounded.

Hold for five to ten deep breaths.

PI-GASM!

Pilates offers another great opportunity to have orgasms! Invest in a Pilates circle (they aren't expensive, maybe around $30, and you can easily find them on the Internet). With your back and head resting on the ground, and your arms outstretched on either side of your body, place the Pilates circle between your knees. Raise up your pelvis, and at the top of the raise, squeeze your muscles all the way from your knees and thighs, down into your pelvic area. Squeeze back from your vaginal canal and add an extra squeeze on the lower third of the V through your thighs and back to your knees. Repeat thirty times before masturbation or sex.

198

Pleasure Checklist

Here are some fun suggestions to get you and your partner geared up for passion. What else can you add?

_____Go on a date and don't wear any underwear.

_____Put yourself in your favorite sexual position while still wearing your clothes to remind your partner just how you like it.

_____Cut out the pockets out of a pair of jeans, and while you're out on town, have your partner reach for something in your pocket.

_____Buy an erotic DVD and watch it with your partner.

_____Buy some erotic literature and read a passage to your partner.

_____Have your partner read a passage of erotic lit to you.

_____Bring your partner to orgasm using only your hands.

_____Have your partner bring you to orgasm, hands only.

_____Bring your partner to orgasm using your mouth.

_____Have your partner bring you to orgasm with their mouth.

_____Explore a sex shop and bring home a toy that you would both like to try.

_____Make dinner in something ultra sexy.

_____Take a bath together and stimulate each other under the bubbles.

GETTING IT *down*

Here's your very own checklist to orgasm. Go through the activities listed. Once you've tried something, check it off the list. And don't stop till you've gone through the whole list. When you do have an orgasm, take notes on how you got there.

These notes (sexual journals) are important to remind you of how you sexually function and what brings you to orgasm. You can also share this information with your partner so she knows exactly what you like.

1. Pull out a mirror and get to know your vulva. Write down what it looks like.

   _____

   _____

2. Do you like how it looks? What do you like about it?

   _____

   _____

3. Is there anything you don't like? Why?

   _____

   _____

   _____

4. Stimulate your clitoris, but don't have a goal in mind. Only do what feels good. Record what you did.

   _____

   _____

   _____

5. Go on a mission to find your G-spot. Now stimulate your G-Spot with the techniques we covered earlier (see page 78). Do what feels good. Record what you did.

_____

_____

_____

_____

6. Try a combination of clitoral and G-Spot stimulation. What works and why?

_____

_____

_____

7. Stimulate yourself thinking of a favorite sexual fantasy. What moment was it in your fantasy that pushed you right over the edge?

_____

_____

_____

_____

8. Experiment with a sex toy, like a bullet vibe or Hitachi magic wand. Write down the sex toy used, what feels good about it, and why it feels good.

_____

_____

_____

9. Write down any techniques you tried that didn't work.

_____

_____

_____

10. Have your partner pleasure you using the oral and manual techniques we covered earlier in this book. List the techniques and what you liked or didn't like about them. (This can inspire you to create some of your own!)

_____

_____

_____

_____

_____

_____

closing THOUGHTS

I want to leave you with this really cool quote from a book called *The Multi Orgasmic Couple* because it's a sentiment I truly believe in and try to live: "Once you can have as many orgasms as you wish, you are able to realize that the orgasmic pulsations themselves are simply part of a continual process of harmonizing with you and your partner and with the world."

My wish for every one of you, for every woman on the planet, is to be able to have orgasms as easily and frequently as possible.

I may be an expert on sex and orgasms today, but like most of you, I didn't start out that way. Growing up, I wasn't taught that much about sex at all and I didn't have a clue what an orgasm was. I actually stumbled upon my first orgasm in my twenties, and it was definitely something I wanted to repeat again and again and have found all kinds of ways to enjoy orgasms.

This is the book I could have used way back when, and I hope it's been helpful for you now. In fact, I hope you've found it informative enough that you'll pass it on to another woman you know who could use a little more **Vitamin O** in her life!

Please feel free to send me an e-mail if you have any questions at drnatashat@aol.com, and please visit me online regularly at **www. drnatasha.com.**

ACKNOWLEDGMENTS

This book wouldn't be possible without my husband Charlie Solomon Jr., Dr. Tony Cahill, Carty Talkington, Virginia McAlester, Jennifer Griffin and Sharon Bowers of the Miller Agency, Skyhorse editors Ann Triestman and Kristin Kulsavage, the Institute for Advanced Study of Human Sexuality, Ted McIlvenna, Gomez, Gomu, and the extraordinary Francine LaSala. Thank you so much.

RESOURCES

Adam and Eve
Toys for women and men, DVDs, and other products.
(800) 293-4654
adamandevetoys.com

Babeland
Toys for women and men, DVDs, and more.
(800) 658-9119
babeland.com

Coco de Mer (also in the UK)
Designer sex toys and lingerie; specialized leather goods; erotic housewares and accessories; erotic books and movies; erotic jewelry and more.
8618 Melrose Avenue
Los Angeles, CA 90069
310 652 0311
cocodemerusa.com

Come As You Are (Canada)
A cooperatively run sex toy, book, and DVD store.
701 Queen Street West
Toronto, Ontario M6J 1E6, Canada
(877) 858-3160
comeasyouare.com

Condoms To Go
5315 Greenville Avenue
Dallas, Texas
214-368-2470
condomstogousa.com

Eve's Garden
evesgarden.com

Forbidden Fruit
Sex toys, costumes, and other adult products, workshops, and more.
108 East North Loop Blvd.
Austin, TX 78751
800 315-2029
forbiddenfruit.com

Good Vibrations
Sex toys, DVDs and video on demand, books, and more.
Several store locations in the San Francisco area.
(800) BUY-VIBE
goodvibes.com

KiKi De Montparnasse
79 Greene Street, New York 10012
kikidm.com

RESOURCES

Larry Flynts Hustler Hollywood
DVDs, books, magazines, sex toys, and more.
hustlerhollywood.com

Sara's Secret
810 North Central Expressway
Plano, Texas
972-578-6661
sarassecret.com

Shades of Love
300 W Bitters Rd # 150
San Antonio, Texas 78216-1690
(210) 494-3006
theshadesoflove.com

The Pleasure Chest
Located in New York, Chicago and Los Angeles
Thepleasurechest.com

TULIP
1422 Milwaukee Avenue
Chicago, IL 60622
773.227.7575
mytulip.com

Xandria Collection
xandria.com

ABOUT
THE
AUTHOR

D r. Natasha is the author of *A Little Bit Kinky* and a certified clinical sexologist with a doctorate in human sexuality. With nearly twenty years of experience in a thriving practice, she's coached tens of thousands of people to have more fulfilling sex lives. She's been a nationally syndicated radio host and a guest on thousands of radio and TV shows worldwide. She has directed, produced, and successfully marketed twenty-three sex self-help DVDs, which have sold more than 100,000 copies, and has conducted numerous sexuality seminars. Dr. Natasha was featured in a *Playboy* "Women of the Internet" pictorial, and her advice has appeared in numerous publications, including *Cosmo, Men's Health, Glamour, Woman's Own, Hustler,* and *The National Enquirer.* A member of ASECT (American Association of Sexuality Educators, Counselors and Therapists) and SSSS (The Society for the Scientific Study of Sexuality), she divides her time between Dallas and L.A .